Everyday
LOW-LECTIN
Cookbook

More than 100 Recipes for Fast and Easy Comfort Food for Weight Loss and Peak Gut Health

—

CLAUDIA CURICI

HARVARD
COMMON
PRESS

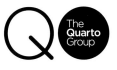

Inspiring | Educating | Creating | Entertaining

Brimming with creative inspiration, how-to projects, and useful information to enrich your everyday life, Quarto.com is a favorite destination for those pursuing their interests and passions.

Library of Congress Cataloging-in-Publication Data

Names: Curici, Claudia, author.
Title: Everyday low-lectin cookbook : fast and easy comfort food for weight
  loss and peak gut health / Claudia Curici.
Description: Beverly, MA : The Harvard Common Press, 2023. | Includes
  index. | Summary: "The Everyday Low-Lectin Cookbook offers more than
  fifty recipes for healthier spins on comfort food. Beautiful photos
  accompany these fast and easy comfort food recipes for weight loss and
  peak gut health, written by expert and pioneer of the lectin-free social
  media scene Claudia Curici"-- Provided by publisher.
Identifiers: LCCN 2022023362 | ISBN 9780760377338 (trade paperback) | ISBN
  9780760377345 (ebook)
Subjects: LCSH: Gastrointestinal system--Diseases--Diet therapy--Recipes. |
  Comfort food. | Quick and easy cooking | Weight loss. | Plant lectins. |
  LCGFT: Cookbooks.
Classification: LCC RC819.D5 C868 2023 | DDC 641.5/63--dc23/eng/20220629
LC record available at https://lccn.loc.gov/2022023362

Design: The Quarto Group
Cover Image: Claudia Curici
Page Layout: Sporto
Photography: Claudia Curici

Printed in China

Dedication

To my parents, my husband and my late grandma.
I am forever grateful for all that you've taught me, for supporting me these
past two years, for believing in me. Thank you for always giving me honest feedback
on my food, even if it was not always what I was hoping. Thanks to your filter,
the recipes I share with the world are more likely to be loved by everyone,
not only those on a lectin-free diet.

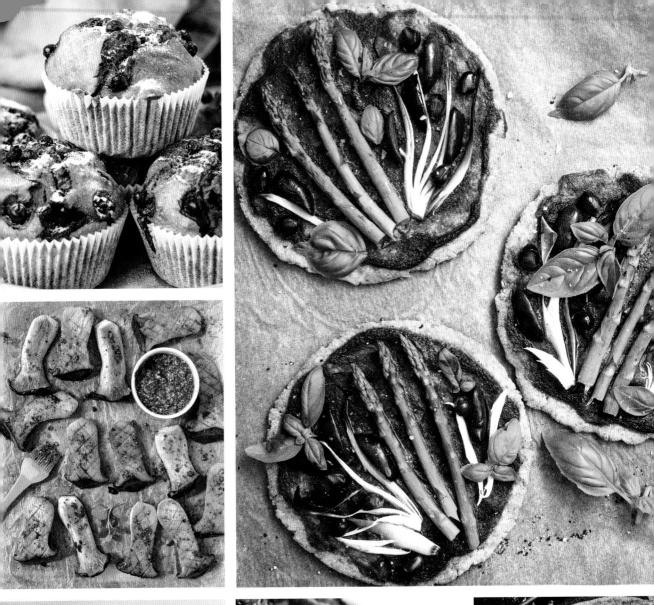
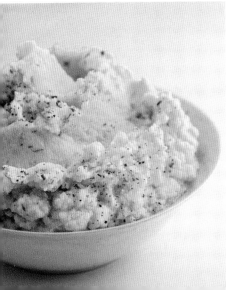
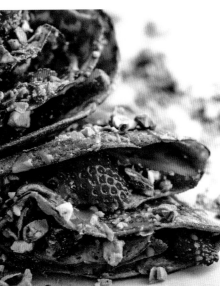
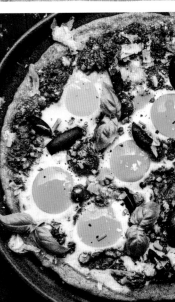

Contents

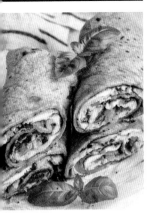

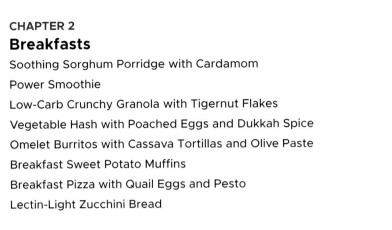

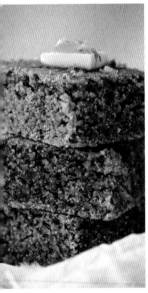

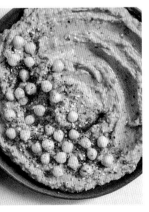

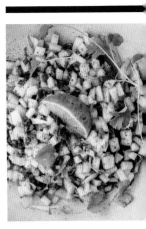

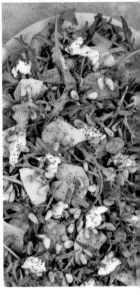

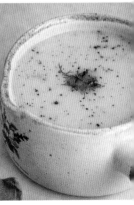

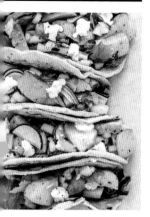

CHAPTER 9

Main Courses with Chicken or Turkey   123

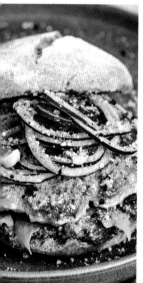

CHAPTER 10

Main Courses with Beef, Lamb, or Pork   139

CHAPTER 11

Vegetable Sides and Vegetarian Mains   151

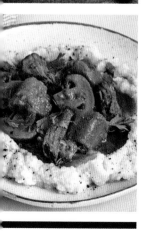

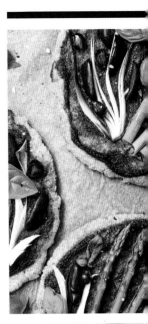

CHAPTER 12
Sweets and Treats

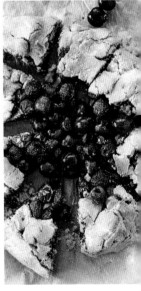

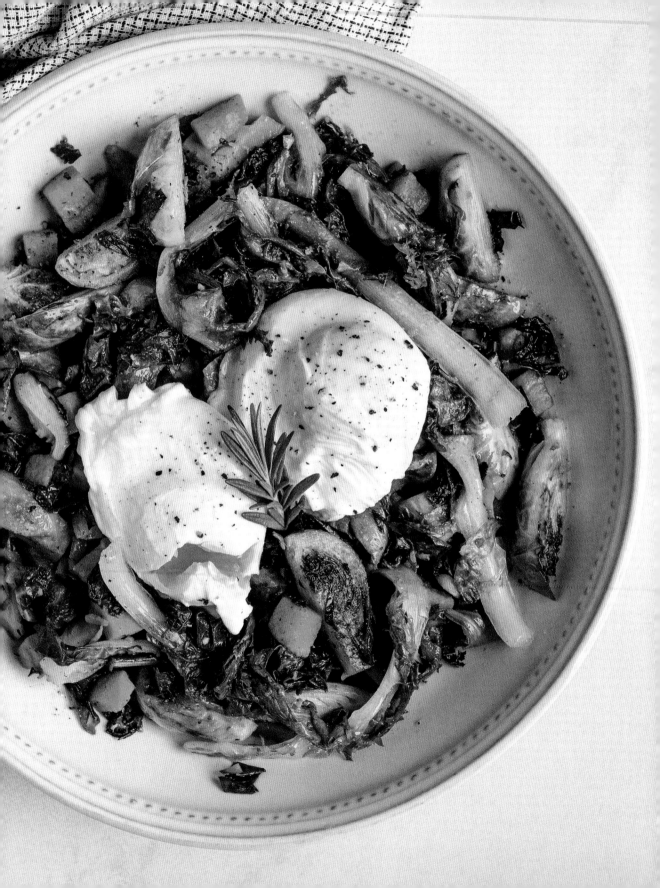

Introduction: The Low-Lectin Revolution

While this book will inevitably serve an audience that has decided to embark on an elimination diet—the elimination of lectins—I don't consider it strictly a diet cookbook. The recipes here were not created from a sense of lacking or deprivation, but as a celebration of hundreds of foods that are neglected in the standard Western diet.

All my recipes were born from a love for nature and the foods she provides and from the desire of nourishing myself and my loved ones with real, healthy foods. Curiosity and a sense of abundance is what drives me, and I hope it will be the same for you.

I developed these recipes over the course of two years while living in Dallas, in the United States—our adoptive country for five years; in Denmark—my husband's native country; and in Romania—my native country. No food was wasted in the making of this book.

The primary purpose behind the creation of these recipes was my and my family's nourishment and the photographs are usually taken before eating, so the food you see in pictures ended on the table and, of course, in our tummies.

The recipes that made it to the book are not only the ones that I loved the most, but those that were also successful with family members and friends. I hope these dishes make your life easier, healthier, and meals with your family more fun.

HOW IT ALL STARTED

In August 2017, after a series of health anxieties, I came across an interview with Dr. Steven Gundry, talking about the impact of lectins in so-called healthy foods on our health. While I never embraced a diet program before, this one resonated with me because I felt I was eating clean and had a healthy lifestyle, but it didn't work for me.

Reading about lectins was like the missing puzzle piece. It made so much sense to me that I decided to give it a try. I haven't looked back since.

People ask me how I manage to stay so focused and dedicated to this lifestyle, and my answer is that I never want to go back to how I was feeling before. In my case, the benefits were so mind-blowing and quick, that for the first time, I felt empowered to improve my health, quality of life, and longevity.

While I wasn't a special cooking talent, I did like cooking, and I was very curious about all the ingredients and foods I had never heard about or considered before. I learned something new about my body and about food every day. I experimented with new ingredients, and I started to pay more attention to where our food comes from and how is it made.

This is how I discovered my passion for creating healthy recipes. Combined with my love for photography, communication and marketing, and my sociology background, plus more than a decade of traveling and working around the world, this new passion manifested into a new community: the lectin-free community gathered around my virtual, healthy, and creative kitchen.

I started an Instagram account and a website, Creative in My Kitchen, a platform to share everything I was discovering and learning in my journey. In my quest to inspire people to lead healthier lifestyles, I felt the need to deepen my knowledge related to health and coaching and graduated from the Institute for Integrative Nutrition (IIN) in New York as an integrative nutrition health coach.

The next step was the opportunity to publish my first cookbook—*The Living Well Without Lectins Cookbook*. For those who are familiar with the Plant Paradox Program, my first book covers Phase 1 and Phase 2 of the Plant Paradox Program, which means a stricter lectin-free approach. Phase 1 is the cleanse phase. It lasts for three days and is the most strict. Phase 2 can last as much as you want or need to reach your health goals, and Phase 3 is the reintroduction and maintenance phase.

Phase 3 is the low-lectin phase. High-lectin foods are reintroduced if prepared correctly to reduce their lectin content. This cookbook is the obvious next step to cover all three phases of the Plant Paradox approach.

WHAT IS THE PLANT PARADOX?

The Plant Paradox is a lifestyle guideline created by Dr. Steven Gundry, a renowned cardiologist, the director of the International Heart & Lung Institute in Palm Springs, California, and the founder and director of the Center for Restorative Medicine in Palm Springs and Santa Barbara.

The Plant Paradox is not a fad diet, and it's not addressed to those looking for dramatic, temporary weight loss. While achieving and maintaining a healthy weight is one of the benefits of this program, the Plant Paradox is designed to reduce chronic inflammation overall and to be adopted for life, as an alternative to the standard American diet or any other similar, unhealthy Western lifestyles.

These are, in a nutshell, the principles of the Plant Paradox Program:

- Eat a predominantly lectin-light diet, avoiding foods high in lectins or preparing high-lectin foods to reduce their lectin content.

- Avoid sugar and high-sugar fruits, especially fruits out of season.

- Eliminate highly processed foods from your diet, including industrial seed and vegetable oils.

- Reduce animal protein and make sure the animal protein you eat is high quality, fed a natural diet, and raised sustainably and humanly.

- Avoid endocrine disruptors: broad-spectrum antibiotics, non-steroidal anti-inflammatory drugs known as NSAIDs such as ibuprofen, and stomach acid blockers; artificial sweeteners such as sucralose and aspartame; endocrine disruptors found in household, skin care, and beauty products; air pollution, exposure to mold, arsenic in food, heavy metal exposure, and plastic exposure; GMO foods; Roundup herbicide; and constant exposure to blue light.

WHAT ARE LECTINS?

Lectins are the defense mechanism of plants developed millions of years ago as a way to protect themselves and their offspring from being eaten by insects, animals, and more recently, humans. According to Dr. Gundry, lectins are a long-term defensive strategy, found in all plants, but highly concentrated in only a few.

However, plant-based foods are important for a healthy lifestyle and to maintain health and increase longevity. So, we don't want to avoid plants because of lectins, but to learn how to prepare them to neutralize their anti-nutrients and maximize their benefits.

WHAT ARE THE FOODS WITH A HIGH CONTENT OF LECTINS?

- Grains and pseudo-grains, except for sorghum, millet, fonio, and teff, which are considered lectin-free

- Legumes, beans, and soy

- Nightshades: tomatoes, potatoes, peppers, eggplant, and goji berries

- Pumpkins, melons, cucumbers, and zucchini

- Almond skins, peanuts, and cashews

- Pumpkin seeds, sunflower seeds, and chia seeds

- Industrially raised and produced animal protein

HOW DO LECTINS AFFECT US?

Lectins are large, sticky proteins that will bind to sugar and try to damage the mucosal lining of your gut. A healthy gut can withstand a certain amount of lectin attack, but if your diet is heavy in lectins and your gut is already damaged from an unhealthy lifestyle, the lectins will trigger the production of a protein called zonulin, which will make holes in your gut wall.

Ever heard of "leaky gut syndrome?" Pieces of bacteria will then be allowed to enter your bloodstream and lymphatic system, triggering your immune system, which will result in widespread inflammation and set the stage for autoimmune diseases.

According to Dr. Gundry, avoiding lectins in your diet will remove the root cause of "leaky gut" and give your gut lining a chance to recover.

HOW TO MAKE HIGH-LECTIN FOODS COMPATIBLE WITH A LECTIN-LIGHT DIET

While a stricter lectin-free approach may be required at the beginning of your healing journey, it is possible to reintroduce high-lectin foods if they are prepared in ways to reduce their lectin content. However, this should be a personal approach, and reintroductions should be done gradually to understand how each food affects us.

There are a few ways to remove lectins in your favorite vegetables:

1. Soaking and pressure cooking
2. Removing peels and seeds
3. Fermentation

This is an overview of the categories of foods that can be reintroduced and the appropriate preparation method.

Tomatoes, peppers, and eggplant

These are on the list of nightshade vegetables, but they are technically fruits. Removing the peels and seeds from these foods will eliminate most of the harmful lectin content. Even so, some people will still be highly sensitive to nightshades. It is best to consume these foods while in season and in moderation. Fermentation and pressure cooking are also a great method to reduce lectins in night-shades.

White potatoes

White potatoes should be pressure cooked and allowed to cool in the refrigerator, preferably overnight, before consuming. This way, the resistant starch content will increase.

Squashes, zucchini, and cucumbers

Remove the peels and seeds. Consume in season and in moderation.

Beans and legumes

Soaking overnight, changing the water several times, and pressure cooking will considerably lower the lectin content in these foods. Consume in moderation.

Rice: Indian basmati rice, red rice, and black rice

Pressure cook and allow to cool overnight in the refrigerator before reheating or consuming.

Wheat

While consuming wheat is not recommended, the healthiest way to do it is to eat slow fermented bread (real sourdough), made with ancient and organic types of wheat. A real bread will only have three ingredients: flour, water and salt.

A LECTIN-LIGHT PANTRY

There is a famous Internet meme: "I start my diet when I get rid of all the stuff I already have in my pantry." Unfortunately, this pretty much means never. The very first step when embracing a new lifestyle is cleaning out your pantry. Get rid of everything that is on the NO list and start filling it with only compliant items.

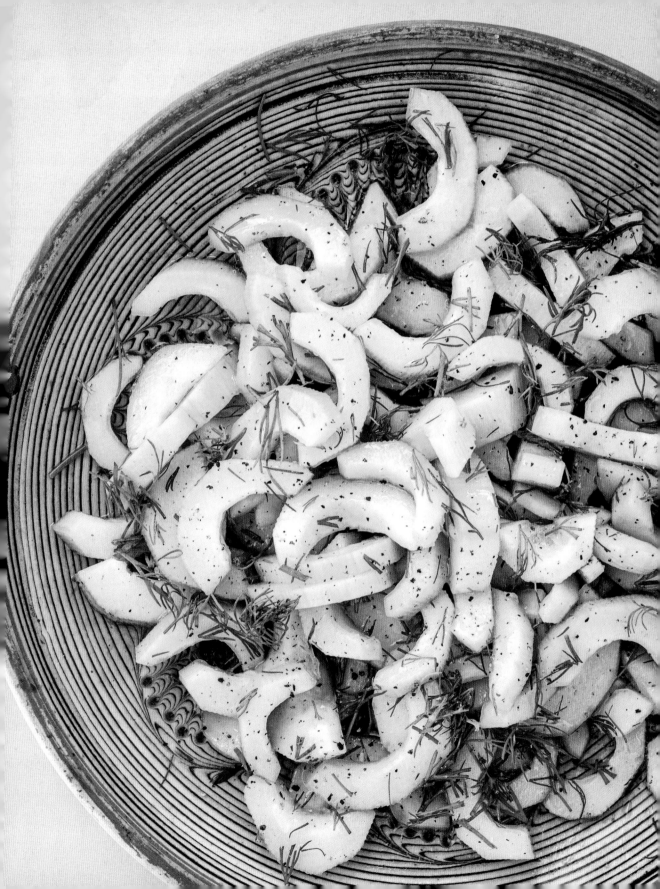

PANTRY ITEMS THAT NEED PRESSURE COOKING

A pressure cooker is one of the most important cooking tools you need in your kitchen. With the help of a pressure cooker, you can reduce lectins in many lectin-heavy foods, especially beans, legumes, and nightshades.

IMPORTANT NOTE: *While I'm giving you some instructions on how to pressure cook certain foods, the instructions from your manual are always the most appropriate and safe. There are many types of pressure cookers around the world, and I know a lot of people are familiar with the Instant Pot, but they don't all work the same as an Instant Pot. Even the different brands of electric pressure cookers work differently.*

WARNING: Never fill your pressure cooker with more liquid or content than allowed as per the user's manual. Follow the instructions in the manual that comes with your pressure cooker.

Beans and legumes

When it comes to beans, I always soak them overnight, change the water several times, and then pressure cook them with about double the quantity of water. When they are ready, I discard the water and use the beans in meals or freeze them.

Sometimes, I add rosemary or thyme, a bay leaf, onion, and a carrot for more taste, but it's not necessary. I never add salt when pressure cooking beans.

The best meal preparation advice I can give you is to pressure cook all type of beans in advance and freeze them in individual portions. You can also use canned beans when the cooking option is not available. The canning process involves pressure cooking, but not necessarily soaking. Find a brand that soaks the beans before canning, preferably organic and BPA-free, and always check the rest of the ingredients.

When buying beans, dry or canned, I always go for organic. Chickpeas are especially contaminated with pesticides.

I use different cooking times for different (soaked) beans: 15 minutes for adzuki and lima beans, 25 minutes for garbanzo and black beans, and 30 minutes for white beans. I pressure cook green lentils for 9 minutes, but usually don't soak them. Other types of lentils, like yellow or red lentils, will go mushy when pressure cooked. They need less time, and they are more appropriate for creamy soups or stews. It is best to follow the instructions in the booklet that comes with your pressure cooker.

Potatoes

Pressure cooking will remove some of the lectins in white potatoes, but it is recommended that potatoes are only consumed after cooling overnight. While I use potatoes in warm dishes occasionally, the best way to enjoy their nutrients and resistant starch properties is in the form of a cold potato salad.

I pressure cook medium-size potatoes for 6 minutes, with 2 cups (475 ml) of water, let them cool overnight, and use them the second day to make salads. For special occasions, I cut or gently smash them and roast them with olive oil, rosemary, and lots of garlic.

Rice

The types of rice approved on a lectin-light diet are Indian basmati rice, black rice, and red rice. They need to be pressure cooked to remove lectins, but they also need to be cooled overnight in the refrigerator and reheated to increase resistant starch content and to lower glycemic response.

Since pressure cookers are all different, it is best to follow the timings and ratios recommended in your cooker's manual.

THE FOUR LECTIN-FREE GRAINS

While these grains don't need to be pressure cooked, you can speed up the cooking time by using a pressure cooker. Sorghum takes the longest to cook on the stove (more than 45 minutes), while millet needs pressure cooking if we want a fluffy, couscous-like texture. Fonio and teff are easy to cook on the stove.

Sorghum

You can find it online or in some specialty stores. Sorghum is perfect to replace rice or quinoa in salads or dishes, make risotto, or use as a side dish, and it also makes a great porridge. Since it doesn't have lectins, you can cook it on the stove, but it takes at least 45 minutes to cook. That's why I prefer to precook it in a pressure cooker and then use the cooked grains to make other dishes like risotto and porridge. Store it in the refrigerator for a few days, or you can even freeze it. What is cool about sorghum is that you can make popped sorghum. It looks and tastes exactly like popcorn, but is much smaller. You can now buy sorghum pasta, and sorghum flour is one of my favorite flours to make bread and crackers. You will find sorghum as an ingredient in quite a few of the recipes in this book.

———————

To cook sorghum in the pressure cooker: rinse well 1 cup (200 g) of sorghum and add it to the cooker with 4 cups (950 ml) of water. Pressure cook on high (normal pressure on a stovetop pressure cooker) for 12 minutes. Let the pressure release naturally. If there is still some liquid left, drain it. Fluff with a fork while cooling down.

Millet

Millet is quite popular and easy to find in stores. It can be cooked on the stove or in a pressure cooker. When cooked on the stove, millet tends to get a porridge-like texture, but you can pressure cook it for more of a grainy and fluffy texture. Cooked this way, millet is perfect for salads like tabbouleh or to replace couscous or rice. Getting the creamy texture is important if making porridge or creamy polenta. Millet also comes as flakes, which can be used as a replacement for oats in porridge and cookies.

———————

To cook millet in a pressure cooker: toast 1 cup (200 g) of millet until fragrant, 2 to 4 minutes (use the sauté option if available), add 2 cups (475 ml) of water, and pressure cook for 8 to 10 minutes. Let the pressure release naturally and then fluff with a fork.

Fonio

A much smaller grain, texture-wise, fonio looks a little bit like sugar. Compared to the other three grains, it's the easiest one to cook. It only takes 3 minutes on the stove. You can serve it as a side, make porridge, add to Buddha bowls, or incorporate in vegan meatballs or burgers.

———————

To cook fonio on the stove, you can start by slightly toasting the fonio, add double the amount of water, bring to a boil, and simmer for about 3 minutes. Fluff with a fork.

Teff

I have been working with teff flour for a while, but the grain is a recent discovery. I absolutely love how it works as porridge. Teff is, like fonio, a very small grain, which takes about 15 minutes to cook on the stove as a porridge. Teff also comes in the form of flakes.

———————

To make teff porridge, slightly toast the teff grains for about 2 to 3 minutes, then add three times the amount of water, bring to a boil, and simmer for about 15 minutes until all the water is absorbed and you get a creamy consistency.

A SHOPPING LIST TEMPLATE BASED ON THE PRINCIPLES OF THE PLANT PARADOX

One of the most important tools that helped me understand what and how to eat for a healthy lifestyle was the Plant Paradox Food Pyramid created by Dr. Gundry. So, I like to organize my shopping list on the same principles. This list doesn't only contain foods you can eat, but it also gives an overview on how to build your plate, every day. This is not an exhaustive list, but it contains the most common foods on the Plant Paradox list. Nothing should be rigid when it comes to food, so keep a flexible approach to suit your lifestyle and your particular circumstances.

GENERAL REMINDERS:

- Eat whole foods, eat the rainbow, diversify, and buy organic, local, and sustainable products.

- Stay well hydrated by drinking water.

- Read labels when buying packaged food: foods that seem compliant can have other ingredients that are not.

- We are all different, so find out what works for you. Age, current health status, personal sensitivities, location, genes, health goals, level of physical activity, gender, and more are all factors that make us unique. Take the below list as a guideline and allow for flexibility in your approach.

- The Plant Paradox plate will be abundant with level 1 foods, a small to moderate amount of the protein of your choice, and resistant starches, all generously drizzled with healthy fats.

- This is a guiding document and not an exhaustive list. With a few exceptions, it does not include packaged food brands, as they differ from country to country.

LEVEL 1:

The Base of the Pyramid

Build your plate around these essential foods. Stock up on these items every time you go shopping. Eat the rainbow. Use healthy fats to cook and season all your meals.

HEALTHY FATS:

Extra-virgin olive oil

Grass-fed, organic ghee

Virgin coconut oil

Red palm oil

Perilla oil

Sesame oil

Walnut oil

Pecan oil

Hemp seed oil

Organic canola oil

MCT oil

Flaxseed oil

CRUCIFEROUS AND LEAFY GREENS:

Arugula

Broccoli, broccolini, and broccoli rabe

Cauliflower

Brussels sprouts

Cabbage: red, green, savoy, and napa

Radishes

Bok choy

Swiss chard

Collard greens

Endive, escarole, dandelion, radicchio, purslane, and spinach

Tops of carrots, beets, radishes, sorrel, wild garlic, patience dock, nettle, pigweed, and red orach

OTHER NONSTARCHY VEGETABLES:

Celery

Carrots

Fennel

Jicama

Kohlrabi

Okra

All lettuce

All fresh herbs including basil, mint, parsley, cilantro, dill, thyme, rosemary, sage, oregano, and chives

Sprouts and micro greens

Daikon radishes

Garlic, leeks, onion, scallions, and shallots

Lemons and limes (fruits)

Avocados (fruits)

Artichokes

Asparagus

FERMENTED FOODS:
(A small amount goes a long way)

Miso paste

Sauerkraut

Kimchi

Other fermented vegetables

Sriracha

Tabasco Red Pepper Sauce

Kombucha (careful with high sugar content)

VINEGARS:

Apple cider vinegar

Wine vinegar

Balsamic vinegar

Rice vinegar

OTHERS:

Mushrooms

Sea vegetables

Seaweed

All spices except for chili flakes

LEVEL 2:

Intermittent Fast or Time-Restricted Eating

Give your body a break from digestion. Voluntarily choosing not to eat anything for 12 to 16 hours a day is actually a healthy habit. It's not even that hard. Sometimes, it just means that you stop eating 4 hours before bedtime, which in itself is a healthy habit. Also called time-restricted eating, you can look at fasting this way: try to eat all your calories during an 8-hour window and stay well hydrated.

LEVEL 3:

Okay to Eat a Limited Quantity of These Foods per Meal

NUTS AND SEEDS:

Flaxseeds, freshly ground

Tree nuts, preferably raw or home roasted: walnuts, pecans, pistachios, Brazil nuts, hazelnuts, Pili nuts, and macadamia

Almonds: only without skin (blanched)

Nigella sativa (black cumin seeds)

Sesame seeds

Basil seeds

Coconut, but not coconut water

Hemp seeds

NUT BUTTERS (100%):

Hazelnut butter

Macadamia butter

Hemp seed butter

Coconut butter (also known as manna)

Walnut butter

Pecan butter

Blanched (white) almond butter

Tahini paste (sesame seed butter)

DAIRY ALTERNATIVES:

Almond milk

Hemp milk

Coconut cream and milk

Coconut yogurt

Almond cream cheese and ricotta (such as Kite Hill)

Nutpods creamer, original

STARCHY VEGETABLES:

Beets (mainly raw)

Green plantain

Green bananas

Sweet potatoes

Yams of all kinds

Root vegetables: parsnip, rutabaga, celeriac (celery root), turnips, and taro

Yucca root (cassava)

Sunchokes

Legumes and beans including lentils, black beans, and adzuki beans: soaked overnight and pressure cooked (Phase 3)

OTHERS:

Cacao powder

Hemp powder

Dark chocolate (80% and above), no dairy, 1 ounce (28 g) per day

LEVEL 4:

Enjoy in Moderation (a Small Quantity, a Few Times a Week)

ANIMAL-SOURCED PROTEIN (2 to 6 ounces [55 to 170 g] per day):

Pastured or omega-3 eggs

Pasture-raised poultry

Wild-caught sustainable fish and shellfish, fresh, frozen, or canned: choose fish low in mercury

FRUITS (IN SEASON):

All berries

Pomegranate

Fresh figs

Apples

Stone fruits: cherries, plums, peaches, and nectarines

Green pears

Green bananas

Green mangoes

Green papaya

Other fruits in season

FLOURS:

Nut flour: blanched almond flour (not almond meal), hazelnut, chestnut, acorn, etc.

Coconut flour

Cassava flour

Tigernut flour

Cauliflower flour

Sweet potato flour

Arrowroot flour

Tapioca flour

Flaxseed meal

Psyllium husk flakes

Sorghum flour

Teff flour

Millet flour

NIGHTSHADES & CUCURBITS:

NOTE: Some people can still have a high sensitivity to these foods, so use ONLY IN PHASE 3.

Tomatoes, peppers, cucumbers, zucchini, pumpkins, and eggplant, if peels and seeds are removed and/or pressure cooked

Potatoes only after cooled in the refrigerator, mainly when they are available locally and organically grown

GRAINS:

Millet

Sorghum

Teff

Rice: Indian basmati, black rice, and red rice (pressure cooked and cooled overnight before reheating and eating)

SWEETENERS:

Inulin

Honey, local or manuka (raw)

Erythritol

Monk fruit: granulated or syrup

Yacon syrup

Stevia

Allulose

LEVEL 5:

Eat/Drink a Very Limited Quantity (1 to 2 Times a Week)

RED MEAT:

Grass-fed, grass-finished (also labeled as 100% grass-fed) beef

Grass-fed lamb, bison, and wild game

Heritage and pasture-raised pork

ALCOHOL:

Red wine (preferably high altitude, max 6 ounces [170 g] per serving)

Dark spirits (1 ounce [28 g] per serving)

Champagne (max 6 ounces [170 g] per serving)

DAIRY:

French and Italian butters or local butters made with A2 milk (from grass-fed Guernsey and Jersey cows)

Buffalo mozzarella

Organic cream cheese

South European cheeses or any cheese made with A2 cow, buffalo, goat, and sheep milk (1 ounce [28 g] per serving)

A2 yogurt (4 ounces [115 g] per serving)

Organic sour cream

11 TIPS TO MAKE HOME COOKING EASIER

When it comes to meal prepping and organizing, there are a few things I do to make my life easier and make sure I can always cook something healthy for me and my family. Your pressure cooker and your freezer will be your best friends.

1 **Batch cook and prepare high-lectin foods** and freeze or store in the refrigerator. This way, I have these staples ready to use. I'm referring here to all kind of beans and lectin-free grains.

2 **Batch cook and freeze** bread, tortillas, gnocchi, and sweet treats so you always have something ready to use for a quick meal.

3 **Batch cook chicken** (like a whole chicken) and shred and freeze in individual portions to always have ready to add to meals.

4 **Batch cook soups and stews.** They are easy to freeze and reheat.

5 **After you go to the farmers market or your local store,** wash and dry your vegetables so they are ready to use. To keep greens fresh for a long time, wash and dry with a salad spinner and store them wrapped in paper towels inside plastic or silicon bags. This step will not only save you time but will make the food preparation process more enjoyable.

6 **Use a shortcut when you can.** Canned beans are pressure cooked, and some brands are soaked, organic, and BPA free. Find out which brands in your area follow all these steps and make sure you have these cans in your pantry for emergency use. Also, I think prewashed greens are the best thing ever invented. If you are a busy person, use this shortcut. Try to find compliant brands in your area or in online stores: pesto, mayonnaise, tortillas, lectin-free pasta, jarred roasted peppers, jarred artichokes, olives, and so on.

7 **Check the freezer aisle of your supermarket.** You can find frozen okra, artichoke hearts, avocado, broccoli, spinach, and so much more. The convenience of throwing a bag of frozen veggies in a pan when you are in a rush can't be beaten.

8 **Fill your pantry and refrigerator with all the lectin-light staples:** lectin-free grains and flour, nuts, approved sweeteners, canned food and pasta, a variety of good-quality spices, extra-virgin olive oil, balsamic vinegar, apple cider vinegar, Sriracha, miso, Tabasco Red Pepper Sauce, and more.

9 **Salt makes food taste good and brings out the natural flavors in other ingredients,** even the sweet ones. Always have a few varieties of salt in your pantry: Himalayan pink salt, sea salt, sea salt flakes, iodized sea salt, smoked sea salt, and noniodized salt for fermenting vegetables.

10 **Meatballs, meat patties, and meat loafs are my favorite foods to freeze.** When you cook them, make big batches and freeze in individual portions. You can serve them with salads, with tortillas, with eggs for breakfast, and with pasta or roasted vegetables.

11 **Kitchen tools make cooking easier, and I have my favorites:** a pressure cooker, a blender, a food processor, a mandolin, a salad spinner, and you will be surprised, but a ceramic coated waffle maker can make your life so easy. Mix compliant flours, eggs, and flavorings, even vegetables, and use a waffle maker to cook them. I think it's easier than making pancakes.

HOW TO USE THIS COOKBOOK

- Cook breads, sauces, pestos, meatballs, and meat loafs in batches and freeze. In fact, most of the recipes in this book can be frozen.

- Mix and match. Use the recipes in the Vegetable Sides section to add to a simple grilled fish or chicken. Use a side from one dish with another protein of your choice.

- Season to your own taste. Some of us like more salt, some more sour, some love strong herb flavors, and some prefer milder flavors. Always taste the food while you are preparing and adjust spices and flavorings to suit your family's taste.

- Cook sweet treats, granola, even pancakes and waffles in batches, portion, and freeze. Whenever the sweet tooth hits you, take something out. There are always cookies and cakes in my freezer.

- Allow for flexibility and creativity. Don't get stuck if you don't have one ingredient, especially when it comes to main courses or sides. Replace the missing ingredients with something similar you have.

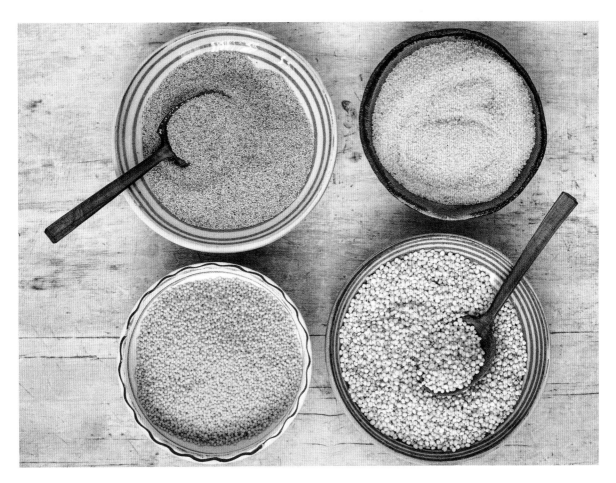

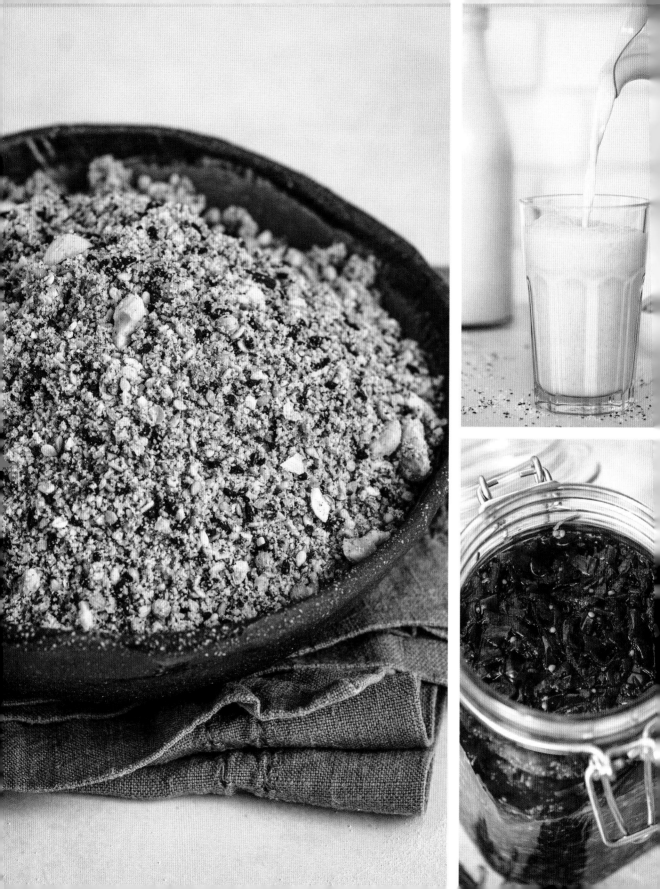

1

Basics

Clockwise from top left: Dukkah, Spice, and Nut Mix (page 28); Homemade Hemp Milk (page 33); Sauerkraut with Red Cabbage and Carrots (page 32)

27

DUKKAH SPICE AND NUT MIX

A variation of a traditional Egyptian spice and nut mix, this dukkah is a staple in our home. I make a big batch in advance, store it in glass jars in the refrigerator, and add it to everything: eggs, salads, yogurt, crackers, bread, and more.

Preparation time:
20 minutes

Makes:
1½ cups (192 g)

½ cup (68 g) roasted hazelnuts, skins removed

¼ cup (36 g) sesame seeds

3 tablespoons (18 g) black cumin seeds (Nigella sativa)

¼ cup (20 g) coriander seeds

2 tablespoons (12 g) cumin seeds

1½ teaspoons black peppercorns

1 teaspoon sea salt flakes

1. Preheat the oven to 300°F (150°C, or gas mark 2). Add the raw hazelnuts to a baking sheet and roast for about 8 to 10 minutes. Remove from the oven and let them cool down for a few minutes. With the help of a kitchen towel or paper towels, rub the nuts to remove the skins. Set aside.

2. In a large skillet, add the sesame seeds and black cumin seeds. Toast on low heat and stir continuously for about 5 minutes. Remove and let cool.

3. In the same skillet, add the coriander, cumin, and peppercorns and toast for about 5 minutes, stirring frequently. Remove from the heat.

4. When all the ingredients have cooled down, add them to a food processor and pulse a few times until they are roughly ground. Add the sea salt flakes and pulse one more time.

5. Store in jars for a few weeks in a cool pantry or in the fridge.

BASIC MAYONNAISE (Low-Histamine)

Quick mayo made with an immersion blender is all the rage on the Internet, but that involves using whole eggs. I like to make mayonnaise with only egg yolks, both for taste and because uncooked egg white can be very high in histamine. I make it on the spot, when I need it, from one or two egg yolks, using a wooden spoon to mix. I know some don't like the strong olive oil taste, but that's exactly why I love using it. Feel free to use avocado oil instead, which is more neutral.

Preparation time:
8 minutes

Makes:
A little more than ¼ cup (60 g)

1 pastured egg yolk

½ teaspoon Dijon mustard

¼ cup (60 ml) extra-virgin olive oil or avocado oil

1 or 2 teaspoons fresh lemon juice

Salt and freshly ground pepper to taste

1. Try to have all the ingredients at room temperature.

2. Add the egg yolk and mustard to a small bowl and mix with a wooden spoon.

3. Start adding the oil one drop at a time, mixing continuously, only in one direction (clockwise).

4. When you finish adding the oil, add the lemon juice, salt, and pepper, mix, and taste. If you use only olive oil, at first it will taste a bit strong, but some of that taste will fade away.

Add some grated garlic to make aioli; capers, shallot, curry powder, and yogurt for a very basic remoulade; Tabasco Red Pepper Sauce for a spicy mayo; or coconut aminos and roasted sesame seeds for an Asian-inspired salad dressing.

BASIC BALSAMIC VINAIGRETTE

The most basic dressing is always a good idea for your salads and veggie bowls. Make sure you have a good-quality balsamic vinegar, such as aged Modena balsamic vinegar. It makes all the difference.

Preparation time:
3 minutes

Makes:
About ¼ cup (60 ml)

1 teaspoon Dijon mustard

1 tablespoon (15 ml) balsamic vinegar

3 tablespoons (45 ml) extra-virgin olive oil

Optional: ½ teaspoon yacon syrup or local or raw honey

Salt and freshly ground pepper to taste

Whisk everything together in a bowl until an emulsion is formed. Store in the fridge until the salad is ready or use immediately.

QUICK PICKLED DAIKON RADISH

These crunchy pickles can be made with any radish. They are a great addition to any meal and are ready in no time. Make them 1 or 2 hours before you plan to eat to allow enough time to cool down.

Preparation time:
15 minutes

Cooking time:
10 minutes

Makes:
2 cups
(475 ml)

½ daikon radish (2 cups [232 g]), peeled or finely sliced with a mandolin

2 garlic cloves, sliced

¾ cup (175 ml) water

¼ cup (60 ml) apple cider vinegar

1 tablespoon (18 g) salt

1 tablespoon (15 g) inulin powder, (12 g) monk fruit, or another sweetener

Optional: 1 teaspoon yacon syrup

1. Add the daikon radish and garlic to a jar that can hold 2 cups (475 ml) of liquid.

2. Combine the water, apple cider vinegar, salt, and sweetener and warm them until they are all dissolved.

3. If you are using yacon syrup, drizzle it on top of the radish slices and then pour the hot liquid on top of the radishes. Let it cool and refrigerate for at least 30 minutes before eating.

SAUERKRAUT WITH RED CABBAGE AND CARROTS

An essential food item in any kitchen, sauerkraut is actually very easy to make—it just requires a little bit of planning. Make a jar at the end of the week to have sauerkraut for the end of the next week. As with anything, a little goes a long way: a small amount will provide the much-needed good bacteria for your digestive system. I like to add some carrots to it, but it's not necessary. While I love the extra nutrition in red cabbage, you can use white cabbage too. Be aware that it's very important to never use iodized salt when fermenting vegetables.

Preparation time:
20 minutes

Makes:
1 quart
(950 ml)

2 pounds (900 g) vegetables: about 1 small to medium red cabbage and 2 big carrots

2 teaspoons sea salt or Himalayan pink salt (NOT iodized)

Optional: spices for extra flavor (1 or 2 tablespoons [weight will vary] of a mix of any of the following spices: mustard seeds, fennel seeds, peppercorns, coriander seeds, bay leaves, cloves, and allspice berries)

1. Make sure you start with a very clean environment: clean glass jars, clean hands, clean work surface, and clean utensils.

2. Shred the cabbage and grate the carrots, transfer to a bowl, sprinkle with salt, and massage with your hands and squeeze it, breaking down the fibers and enabling them to release as much of the juices as possible.

3. If you are using spices, add them to the bottom of the jar.

4. Stuff the vegetables in the glass jar, pressing down as much as possible, and add any liquid left in the bowl.

5. Add something on top of the jar, like a clean towel, that will allow air to get in.

6. Place the jar with the red cabbage on the kitchen counter and every morning and evening, open it and press down the vegetables with a clean spoon. I like to taste it every day and see how it changes (use a clean spoon and don't double dip).

7. Depending on the room temperature, it can take from 4 to 5 days to 2 weeks to get where you want it to be, but it also depends on your taste. My kitchen was pretty warm, and on the fifth day, I closed the jar and transferred it to the fridge (or a cold pantry).

HOMEMADE HEMP MILK

Hemp milk has always been my favorite nondairy plant milk. But, since we moved from the United States to Europe, it has been impossible to find hemp milk in stores. Luckily, hemp seeds are easy to find. This milk alternative is a staple in our house. I make it often and add it to my lectin-free granola, use it to make golden milk, for baking, in smoothies, with porridge, and even in dairy-free savory dressings and sauces.

Preparation time:
5 minutes

Makes:
2½ cups
(570 ml)

¼ cup (37 g) hemp seeds

2¼ cups (535 ml) filtered water

Optional: salt, pure vanilla extract, or any compliant sweetener to taste

1. Add the hemp seeds to a high-powered blender.

2. Top with filtered water and any optional ingredients and blend until smooth (for about 1 minute).

3. Transfer to a glass bottle or jar, cover, and store in the fridge for 2 to 3 days.

4. If you decide to strain it (not necessary, in my opinion), use a nut milk bag.

5. Shake well before using.

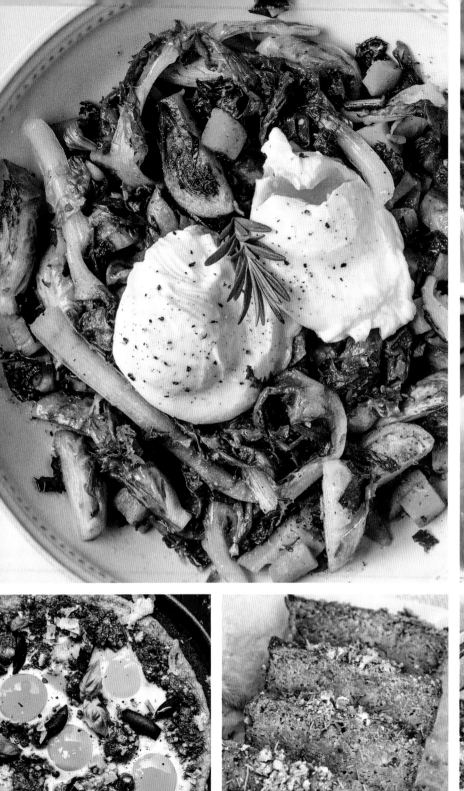
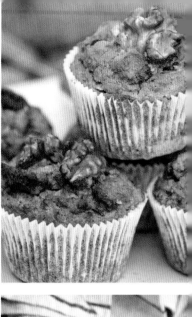
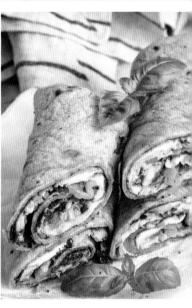
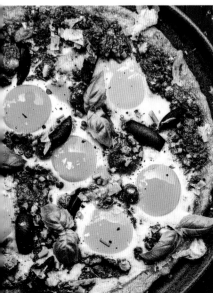
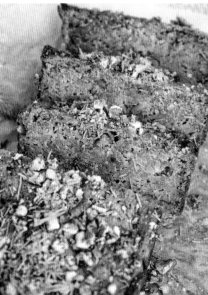
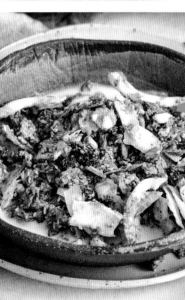

2

Breakfasts

Clockwise from top left: Vegetable Hash with Poached Eggs and Dukkah Spice (page 40); Breakfast Sweet Potato Muffins (page 45); Omelet Burritos with Cassava Tortillas and Olive Paste (page 42); Low-Carb Crunchy Granola with Tigernut Flakes (page 39); Lectin-Light Zucchini Bread (page 48); Breakfast Pizza with Quail Eggs and Pesto (page 46)

SOOTHING SORGHUM PORRIDGE WITH CARDAMOM

This porridge doesn't have many add-ons. It's a soothing meal for when you feel like comfort food, but your stomach can't handle much. Cardamom has antibacterial properties and can help with digestive problems, and I personally love the flavor. If you feel more adventurous, you can get creative with this recipe, like with any porridge. Needless to say, while porridge is usually a morning food, you can eat this any time of the day.

Preparation time:
5 minutes

Cooking time:
10 minutes

Makes:
3 cups (525 g)

2 cups (350 g) cooked sorghum

1 cup (235 ml) hemp milk, homemade (page 33) or store-bought, or another nut milk

1 or 2 cardamom pods, cracked open

½ teaspoon cinnamon

1 tablespoon (15 g) coconut cream

Sweetener to taste: yacon syrup, inulin powder, monk fruit, or local or raw honey

Nut butter

1. Combine the cooked sorghum and hemp milk in a saucepan, add the cardamom and cinnamon and the coconut cream, and simmer until the liquid is absorbed and the consistency becomes creamy, about 5 to 10 minutes.

2. Sweeten with yacon syrup, inulin powder, or monk fruit to your taste. You can also use local or raw honey.

3. Drizzle with nut butter and serve.

COOKING SORGHUM IN THE PRESSURE COOKER:
Rinse well 1 cup (180 g) of sorghum and add it to the pressure cooker with 4 cups (950 ml) of water. Pressure cook on high (normal pressure on a stovetop pressure cooker) for 12 minutes. Let the pressure release naturally. If there is still some liquid left, drain it. Fluff with a fork while cooling down. As always, follow your pressure cooker instruction manual.

POWER SMOOTHIE

This is for those mornings when you don't feel like chewing food. This smoothie is fast to make, and it has enough nutritional value to give you an energy boost in the morning and keep you going until lunchtime. You can adjust the ingredients to fit your taste buds and preferences. If you are not interested in keeping it keto-friendly, adding more blueberries or other berries will increase the sweetness and make it more palatable for children.

Preparation time:
10 minutes

Serves:
4

½ avocado

2 cups (94 g) romaine lettuce (pressed down)

4 tablespoons (39 g) frozen wild blueberries

4 teaspoons (7 g) raw cacao powder

2 teaspoons spirulina powder

1 handful of fresh cilantro

1 tablespoon (15 g) MCT oil

1 teaspoon inulin powder

1 teaspoon yacon syrup

1 cup (235 ml) full-fat coconut milk

1 cup (235 ml) filtered water

Juice of ½ lime

Zest of 1 organic lime, orange, or lemon

Pinch of sea salt

Optional: 1 scoop Vital Reds (Concentrated Polyphenol Blend) dietary supplement or 1 tablespoon (8 g) pomegranate powder

Combine all the ingredients in a high-powered blender. If you feel the need for more sweetness, you can add more yacon syrup or another approved sweetener, more blueberries, or even one scoop of Vital Reds. Serve immediately or store in an airtight container in the fridge, but you should not store it for longer than 12 hours.

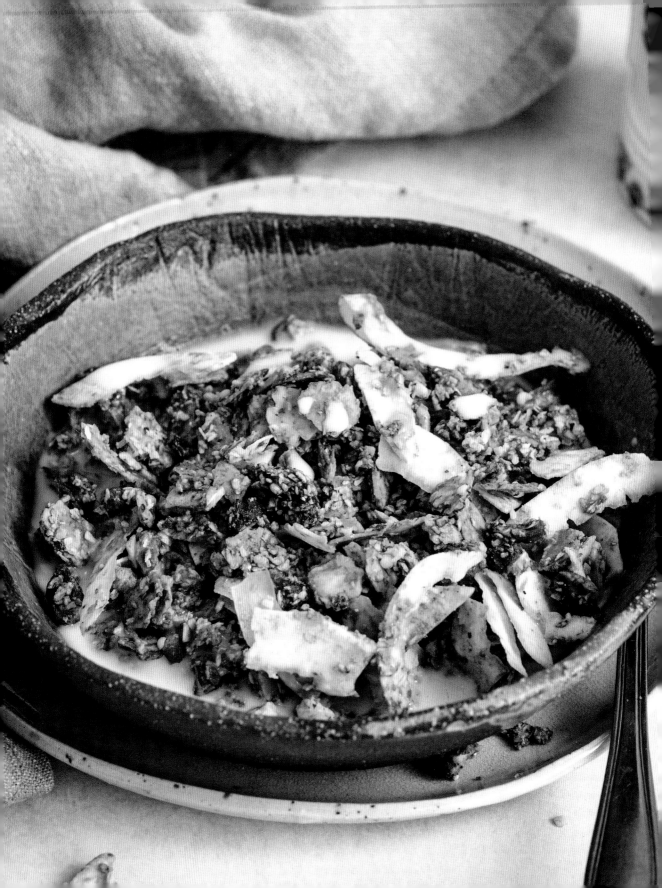

LOW-CARB CRUNCHY GRANOLA WITH TIGERNUT FLAKES

I've always loved homemade granola, and one of the first lectin-free recipes I created was granola, made with green plantain. This time, I used tigernut flakes to make a keto-friendly granola that tastes more like a decadent dessert. Despite the name, tigernuts are tubers, not nuts, and even though they are carbohydrates, they don't raise blood sugar. They also act like a prebiotic. I love to have this granola with cold hemp milk, but it goes well with any type of yogurt.

Preparation time:
15 minutes

Cooking time:
20 minutes

Makes:
About 5 cups
(450 g)

⅔ cup (67 g) raw pecans

½ cup (68 g) hazelnuts (without skin, okay if roasted)

¼ cup (31 g) raw pistachios

3 tablespoons (28 g) hemp seeds

½ cup (40 g) shredded coconut

1 cup (149 g) tigernut flakes

4 tablespoons (56 g) coconut oil

¾ ounce (20 g) dark chocolate (above 80%)

Zest of 1 organic orange

½ teaspoon vanilla powder or 1 teaspoon pure vanilla extract

½ teaspoon sea salt flakes

1 cup (60 g) coconut flakes

1–2 tablespoons (15 to 28 ml) yacon syrup

1. Preheat the oven to 300°F (150°C, or gas mark 2) and prepare a large baking sheet.

2. In a food processor, mix the pecans, hazelnuts, pistachios, and hemp seeds until roughly ground. One or two pulses will be enough. You want to retain some bigger pieces of nuts.

3. Transfer the contents to a mixing bowl. Add the shredded coconut, tigernut flakes, coconut oil, chocolate, orange zest, vanilla, and sea salt flakes and mix well. Don't worry if the coconut oil is solid.

4. Transfer to the oven and bake for 12 to 15 minutes, mixing with a spatula every 5 minutes.

5. After 15 minutes, add the coconut flakes, mix again, and bake for 5 more minutes.

6. Remove from the oven, mix well, drizzle yacon syrup all over the granola, mix again, and let it cool completely (in a cold place if you have space for the baking sheet).

7. Once everything is cold, transfer to glass containers and store in the fridge for up to 5 days or freeze.

VEGETABLE HASH WITH POACHED EGGS AND DUKKAH SPICE

A savory breakfast will give you energy and keep you full and satisfied for a long time. To make a meal like this very easy to prepare, it's beneficial to clean and dry your veggies after you buy them. Also, always having a jar of interesting spice mixes and toppings, like dukkah, will make every meal more flavorful, nutritious, and satisfying. If you don't have a dukkah spice mix, use a zaatar spice mix or simply season with salt, pepper, and cumin.

Preparation time:
10 minutes

Cooking time:
15–20 minutes

Serves:
2

1 small sweet potato, cut into small cubes

8–10 Brussels sprouts, quartered

1 sprig rosemary, cut into 2 pieces

2 garlic cloves, smashed and finely chopped

1 generous handful of Lacinato kale, finely chopped

½ head curly endive or frisée, soaked in cold water for 20 minutes and dried

1–2 tablespoons (15 to 28 ml) extra-virgin olive oil

Salt and freshly ground pepper to taste

2 pastured eggs

2 tablespoons (16 g) Dukkah Spice and Nut Mix (page 28)

1. Prepare all the veggies. If you don't have frisée or curly endive, use any other bitter green, like endive, radicchio, or even romaine lettuce.

2. You need a large sauté pan with a lid. Add a small quantity of olive oil to the cold pan and add the sweet potato and Brussels sprouts. Spread them on the surface of the pan, making sure the Brussels sprouts are cut-side down. Add the rosemary, cover, and start heating on medium heat and cook undisturbed for about 10 minutes. When you start to smell the Brussels sprouts charring, you can take the lid off and check one. You want to get some sear on the cut side. If you see that, you can start tossing everything around.

3. Add the garlic, kale, endive, salt, and pepper and some more olive oil, reduce the heat to low, cover, and cook for 5 more minutes.

4. Take the lid off, stir, and cook for a few minutes more.

5. While the veggies are cooking, heat some water in a deep saucepan. When the water is boiling, turn the heat to the lowest setting, so it doesn't bubble anymore. Crack the eggs into two small coffee cups. Stir the water with a knife or fork, clockwise, and throw one of the eggs in the middle. Once the first egg white sets a little bit, repeat with the second egg. Make sure the water isn't boiling but stays hot. Cover with a lid. It will take about 5 minutes for the egg white to completely set while still having a runny and gooey yolk. Remove with a slotted spoon and place on a paper towel.

6. Add the veggies to a big serving bowl and top with the eggs. Generously sprinkle with Dukkah Spice and Nut Mix and drizzle more olive oil on top.

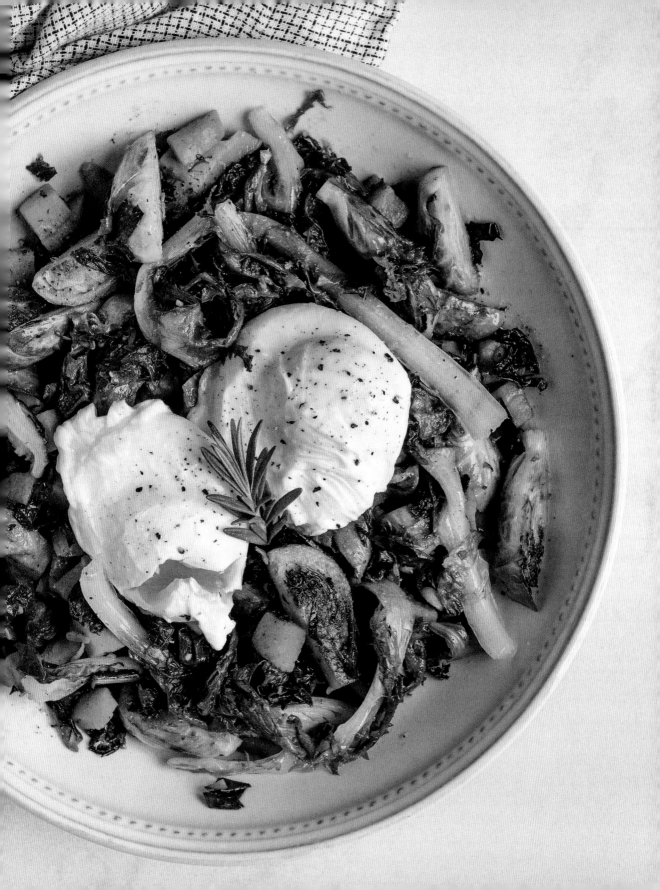

OMELET BURRITOS WITH CASSAVA TORTILLAS AND OLIVE PASTE

A family favorite, these burritos are easy to make and will be loved by kids and adults alike. The cassava tortillas are a staple, and whenever I make a big batch, I store them in the freezer. It only takes a few minutes to thaw and warm them. For these burritos, I recommend bigger-size tortillas, about 10 inches (25 cm). Alternatively, you can use any compliant tortillas you can find in stores (if you live in the United States, that's easy). Feel free to add some compliant cheese. This is a perfect dish for brunch, but who says you can't have it for dinner?

Preparation time:
20 minutes

Cooking time:
15 minutes

Serves:
2

2 cassava tortillas (the size for burritos, about 10 inches [25 cm]), store-bought, or use the recipe for Easy Cassava Flour Tortillas (page 58)

5 Brussels sprouts, finely sliced

4 small button mushrooms, finely chopped

1 shallot, finely chopped

1 small red bell pepper, peeled and deseeded, finely sliced

1 medium heirloom tomato, preferably red, peeled and deseeded

3 pastured eggs

2 tablespoons (28 ml) extra-virgin olive oil

¼ teaspoon salt

⅛ teaspoon freshly ground pepper

2–3 tablespoons (30 to 45 g) olive tapenade, (50 to 75 g) olive paste, or (12 to 18 g) simply chopped Kalamata olives

A few leaves of fresh parsley

A few leaves of fresh basil

Optional: a few drops of Tabasco Red Pepper Sauce or Sriracha for a kick

Optional: compliant cheese such as buffalo or goat cheese

1. Prepare the tortillas. If they are in the freezer, take them out and warm them in a pan or a griddle, making sure they remain soft (if you leave them too long, they'll turn crispy). Have them ready and warm when the omelet is done.

2. Prepare the vegetables. Beat the eggs.

3. Add the olive oil to a nonstick pan (such as cast iron or ceramic) on medium heat. When the oil is hot, add the vegetables, except for the tomatoes, and cook, stirring occasionally, for about 5 to 7 minutes. Arrange the vegetables to cover the bottom of the pan.

4. Pour the beaten eggs on top of the vegetables, without stirring, and add the salt and pepper. If you use a larger skillet, the process will be easier as the eggs will cook faster on top. Use a lid and cook on low heat until the eggs are set. If it takes too long, you can break the omelet and flip it so it gets golden on both sides without overcooking it.

5. Spread the olive paste on the tortillas and add the eggs on top. Spread the chopped tomatoes. Sprinkle on some fresh parsley and pepper and add cheese if using and then roll them like a burrito. Slice in half, garnish with fresh basil, and serve with some hot sauce.

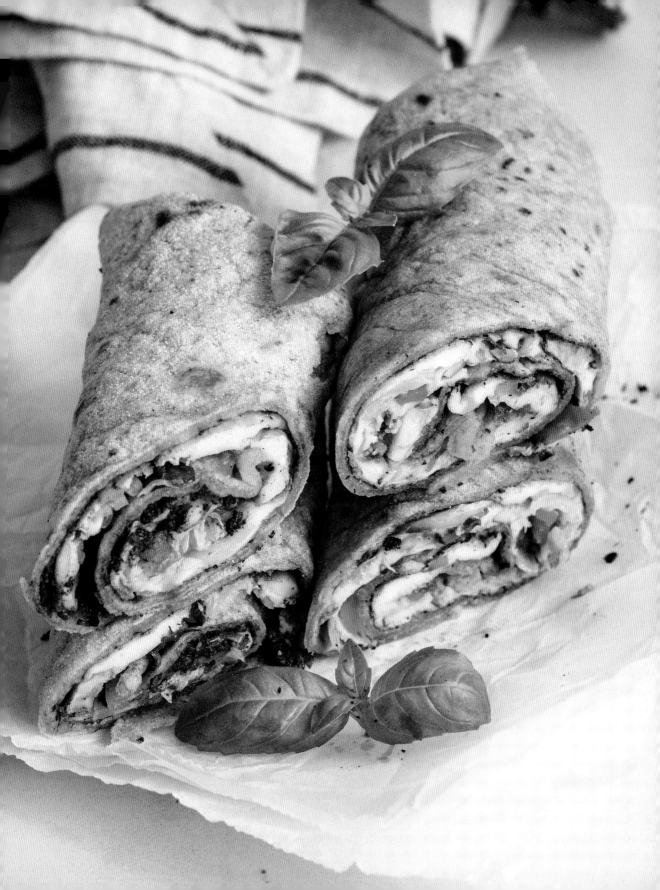

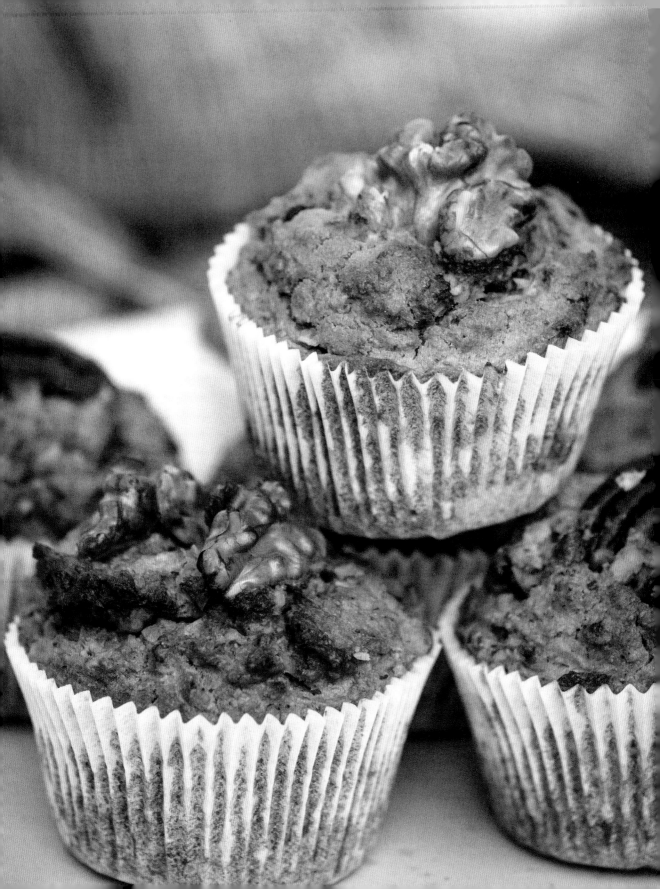

BREAKFAST SWEET POTATO MUFFINS

You know what they say: it's best to avoid breaking your fast with something sweet. But these muffins are made with whole ingredients, have no sugar or sweetener, are rich in healthy fats and protein, and only have a natural sweetness. They are great with coffee or tea, but are also the perfect accompaniment to an egg breakfast or a salad. They can be stored at room temperature for 2 days, stored in the refrigerator for 3 to 4 days, or even frozen.

Preparation time:
20 minutes

Cooking time:
30–35 minutes

Makes:
7 muffins

1 cup (145 g) mixed nuts (walnuts, pecans, and pistachios), plus more for garnish

½ cup (40 g) shredded coconut

Zest of 1 organic lemon

¼ cup (30 g) tigernut flour

¼ cup (35 g) sorghum flour

1 teaspoon baking powder

⅔ cup (219 g) mashed sweet potato

¼ cup (60 g) coconut cream

¼ cup (60 g) extra-virgin olive oil

2 pastured eggs

⅛ teaspoon salt

½ teaspoon cinnamon

½ teaspoon licorice powder

1. Preheat the oven to 350°F (180°C, or gas mark 4). Line a muffin tin with muffin paper liners (makes about seven small muffins).

2. Grind the nuts in a food processor until they resemble the texture of cauliflower rice. It's okay if some pieces are bigger and some smaller. In fact, that's what you are looking for.

3. Mix the ground nuts, shredded coconut, lemon zest, tigernut flour, sorghum flour, and baking powder in a big bowl.

4. In a food processor or blender, combine the sweet potato, coconut cream, olive oil, and eggs until creamy.

5. Add the cream mixture to the dry ingredients, add the spices, and combine with a spatula.

6. Fill each muffin liner with the batter and add half a walnut or pecan on top, gently pushing it into the batter.

7. Bake for about 30 minutes. I used a cake setting, which makes things bake faster, so it might take an extra 5 minutes if you use a normal baking setting. They are ready when golden brown on top and no longer soft to the touch.

8. Let them cool for 10 to 15 minutes before eating.

BREAKFAST PIZZA WITH QUAIL EGGS AND PESTO

Quail eggs are nutritious and really cute, so why not use them more in your diet? I really love this way of baking them on a pizza crust or flatbread, generously layered with pesto, complete with the umami flavor from Parmigiano Reggiano and olives. You can certainly get creative with this concept and add your own spin on it. It's perfect for brunch, but who says you can't have this for dinner? A personal size pizza crust can make two servings if you are eating this for breakfast. But you can double the recipe if you are really hungry. If using store-bought tortillas as a base, layer two on top of each other, as they are pretty thin.

Preparation time:
20 minutes

Cooking time:
8–10 minutes

Serves:
2

1 Super Easy Pizza Crust (7 inches, or 18 cm) (page 54) or use 2 Easy Cassava Flour Tortillas (page 58)

¼ cup (65 g) Asparagus Pesto (page 86), or any pesto you have

6 pastured quail eggs

4–6 chopped olives or olive paste

2 tablespoons (10 g) grated Parmigiano Reggiano

Pinch of dried oregano

Pinch of sea salt flakes

Pinch of pepper

Fresh basil leaves

2 tablespoons (6 g) chopped fresh chives (or ½ teaspoon dried chives)

Optional: a few drops of Tabasco Red Pepper Sauce

1. Preheat the oven to 400°F (200°C, or gas mark 6). If the pizza crust is frozen, first warm it up in the oven. If you are using a tortilla, which is thinner, don't warm it up before (but it needs to be thawed) and use a lower temperature, such as 350°F (180°C, or gas mark 4).

2. Spread a generous layer of pesto on the pizza crust.

3. Carefully crack open the quail eggs with the edge of a knife and arrange them on top of the pesto. Add the chopped olives.

4. Bake on a baking sheet for about 8 minutes or until the egg whites are set.

5. Remove from the oven, sprinkle with grated Parmigiano Reggiano, oregano, sea salt flakes, and pepper, and garnish with fresh basil leaves and a few more drops of fresh pesto. Add the chopped chives and Tabasco Red Pepper Sauce for a kick.

How to Make Basic Pesto
If you don't have any premade pesto on hand and you need to make some on the spot, just blend a generous handful of basil leaves, 2 tablespoons (15 g) pistachio nuts (or [18 g] pine nuts), ¼ cup (60 ml) extra-virgin olive oil, 1 tablespoon (15 ml) fresh lemon juice, and salt and freshly ground pepper to taste. It's that easy.

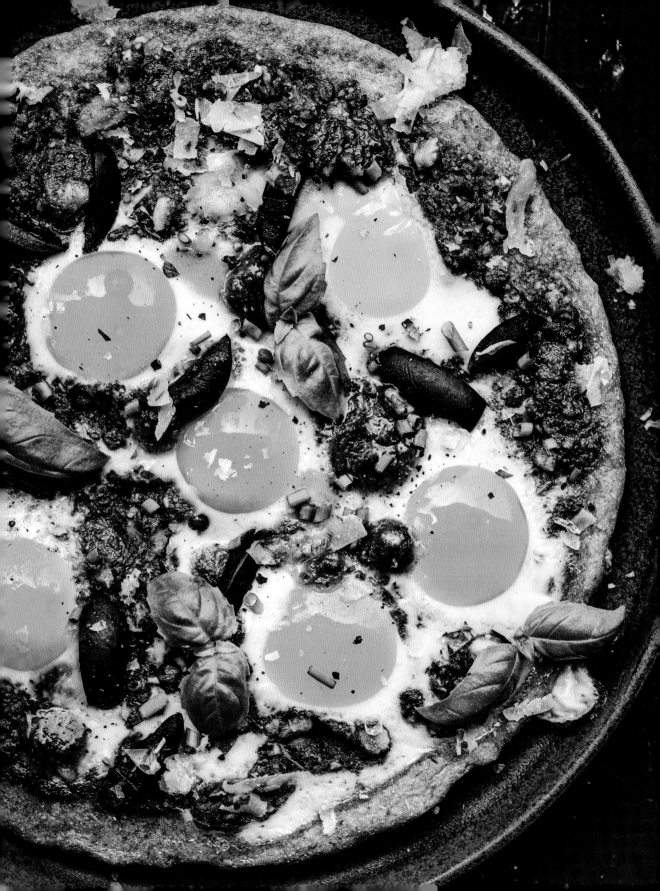

LECTIN-LIGHT ZUCCHINI BREAD

If you thought you would never be able to eat zucchini again, please allow me to be the bearer of good news: you can eat zucchini if you remove the peels and seeds, where the lectins are, and you can certainly use them to make delicious gluten-free, sugar-free zucchini bread that is also lectin-light. This cake is dense and moist, but it has a light bite. If in season (spring) and available, I recommend using spruce tips for an interesting, piney-citrus flavor, but rosemary can also be used.

Preparation time:
30 minutes

Cooking time:
45 minutes

Serves:
12

DRY INGREDIENTS:

¼ cup (25 g) roasted pecans, finely chopped, plus more for decorating the cake

½ cup (70 g) cassava flour

½ cup (52 g) almond flour

½ cup (56 g) chestnut flour

½ cup (60 g) tigernut flour

1 teaspoon baking powder

½ teaspoon salt

1 teaspoon cinnamon

¼ teaspoon nutmeg

WET INGREDIENTS:

⅓ cup (80 ml) extra-virgin olive oil

1 tablespoon (20 g) local or raw honey or sweetener of your choice ([15 ml] yacon syrup, [12 g] monk fruit, or [15 g] inulin powder)

2 pastured eggs

1 teaspoon pure vanilla extract

Zest of 1 organic lemon

½ cup (120 ml) full-fat coconut milk

1½ cups (180 g) grated zucchini, extra liquid squeezed out

Optional: 1 small handful of chopped spruce tips or 1 tablespoon (2 g) chopped rosemary (or less if you don't like a strong rosemary taste)

1. Preheat the oven to 350°F (180°C, or gas mark 4) and line a loaf pan with parchment paper.

2. If you need to toast the pecans, do it while you prepare the ingredients, at 300°F (150°C, or gas mark 2), for no longer than 10 minutes, as they burn fast. Keep an eye on them. Once toasted, you can finely chop them.

3. Mix the dry ingredients in a small bowl.

4. In a bigger bowl, mix the olive oil with the sweetener if using with a whisk. Add the eggs, vanilla, and lemon zest, and whisk until creamy. Add the coconut milk and combine. Add the grated zucchini.

5. Start adding the dry ingredients to the wet ingredients and incorporate it with the whisk or a spatula. Don't overmix.

6. Add the spruce tips or the rosemary if using and the pecans and combine. You will get a thick batter that will be scooped into the loaf pan.

7. Bake at 350°F (180°C, or gas mark 4) for 40 to 45 minutes until golden brown on top and no longer soft to the touch.

8. Remove from the oven and allow it to cool down, top with the rest of the pecans and chopped spruce tips if using, and drizzle with some local or raw honey or yacon syrup.

NOTE: The spruce tips are not essential for this cake, but if you have them, they will add a nice, subtle pine flavor and lots of nutritional value.

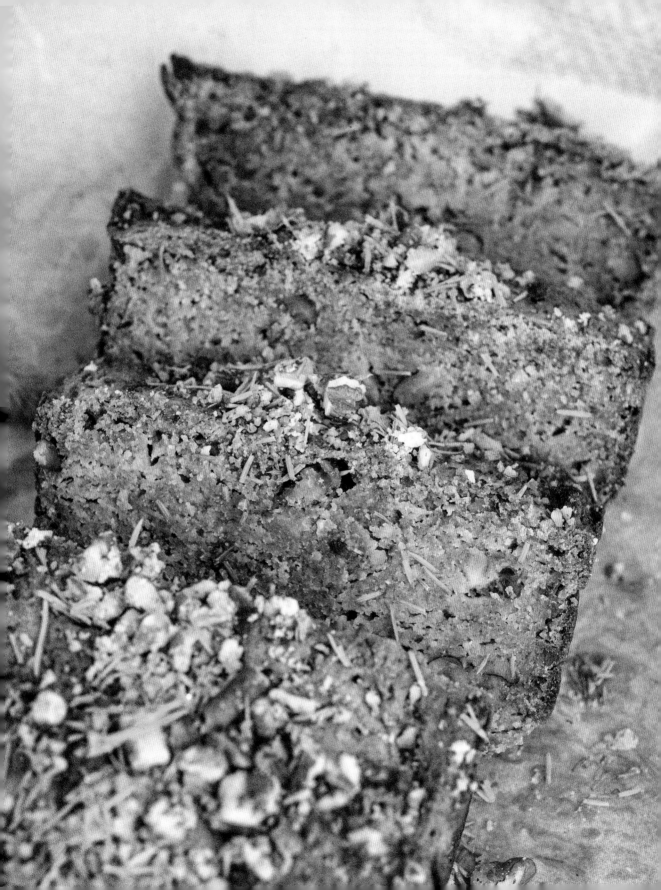

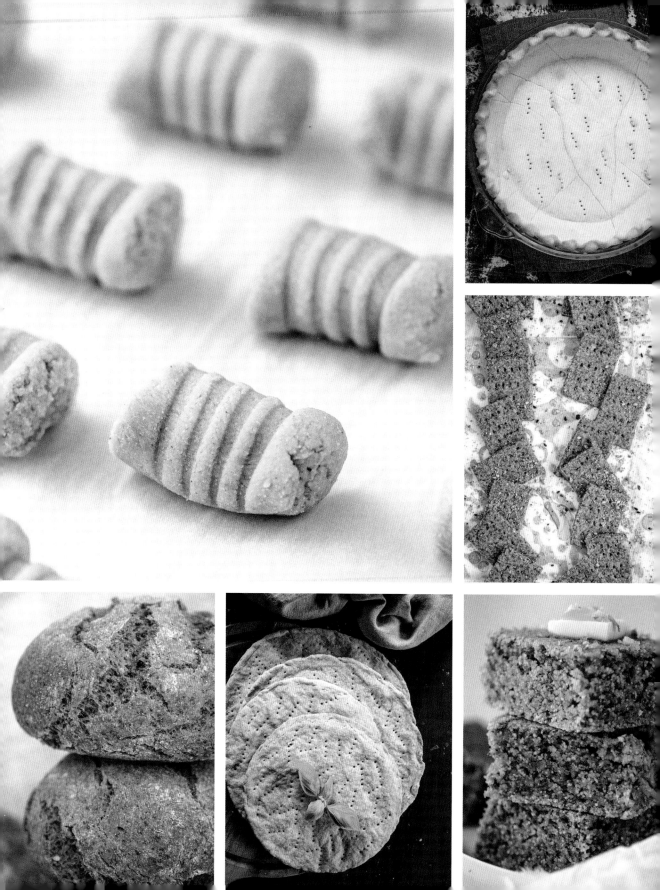

3

Breads, Crackers, Pizza, and Pasta

Clockwise from top left: Green Gnocchi with Arugula and Cassava Flour (page 64); Easy Keto Pie Crust, without Eggs (page 68); Spicy Keto Crackers with Dukkah (page 61); Faux "Corn Bread" with Millet and Walnuts (Page 62); Yucca Root and Sorghum Pizza Crust (page 57); Multipurpose Yeast Dough (hamburger Buns, Dinner Rolls, and Flatbread) (page 52)

MULTIPURPOSE DOUGH
(Hamburger Buns, Dinner Rolls, and Flatbread)

Hamburger buns, dinner rolls, flatbread—this dough can make anything. A friend of mine used this recipe to make a loaf bread. It's very easy to put together, has a light texture and great taste, and can be easily stored. The flatbreads are perfect for the Chicken Gyro Platter with Tzatziki Sauce (page 132), and I use the hamburger buns to make the Turkey Burger with Dukkah Spice Mix and Pesto (page 130). The possibilities are endless.

Preparation time:
35 minutes

Cooking time:
25 minutes

Serves:
6–8

DRY INGREDIENTS:

¾ cup (100 g) cassava flour, plus about ½ cup (70 g)

5 tablespoons (50 g) sorghum flour

5 tablespoons (40 g) tapioca flour

2 teaspoons (10 g) tigernut flour

2 tablespoons (12 g) psyllium husk flakes

1 teaspoon salt

1¾ teaspoons (7 g) dry yeast

1 teaspoon baking soda

Optional: a mix of seeds (about 1–2 teaspoons of each): poppy seeds, sesame seeds, black cumin seeds (Nigella sativa), and hemp seeds

WET INGREDIENTS:

6 tablespoons (90 g) extra-virgin olive oil

3 pastured eggs

1 teaspoon apple cider vinegar

¾ cup (175 ml) lukewarm water

EXTRA:

½ to ¾ cup (70 to 105 g) sorghum flour for kneading and shaping

1. Preheat the oven to 375°F (190°C, or gas mark 5). Prepare a baking sheet, a work surface, and parchment paper.

2. Mix all the dry ingredients in a big bowl. The type of yeast I used had to be mixed with the dry ingredients, but if you use another type, follow the instructions on the package.

3. Whisk the olive oil, eggs, and apple cider vinegar in a smaller bowl.

4. Pour the wet ingredients on top of the flour mixture and combine with a spatula. Start adding the water, gradually, and continue to incorporate the ingredients.

5. Gradually start adding the extra 70 g cassava flour and combine. The dough will thicken but will remain soft and sticky. When it is too thick for the spatula, you can use your hands. After you've added a little less than ½ cup (70 g) of cassava flour, shape the dough into a ball and let it rest for about 40 minutes, covered, in a warm place. This dough doesn't really rise much, so don't worry.

6. When the 40 minutes are done, take the dough out. If making burger buns, split into six equal parts and shape into rounds and gently flatten them. Generously use the extra sorghum flour for kneading and dusting when shaping the dough. Gently knead, but don't overwork the dough. Bake the burger buns for about 25 minutes.

7. If making flatbreads, you can make between six and eight flatbreads. Roll them out with a rolling pin, thicker than you would do with tortillas, always dusting the work surface and your hands with sorghum flour. Bake for about 12 to 15 minutes. Don't let them dry out too much.

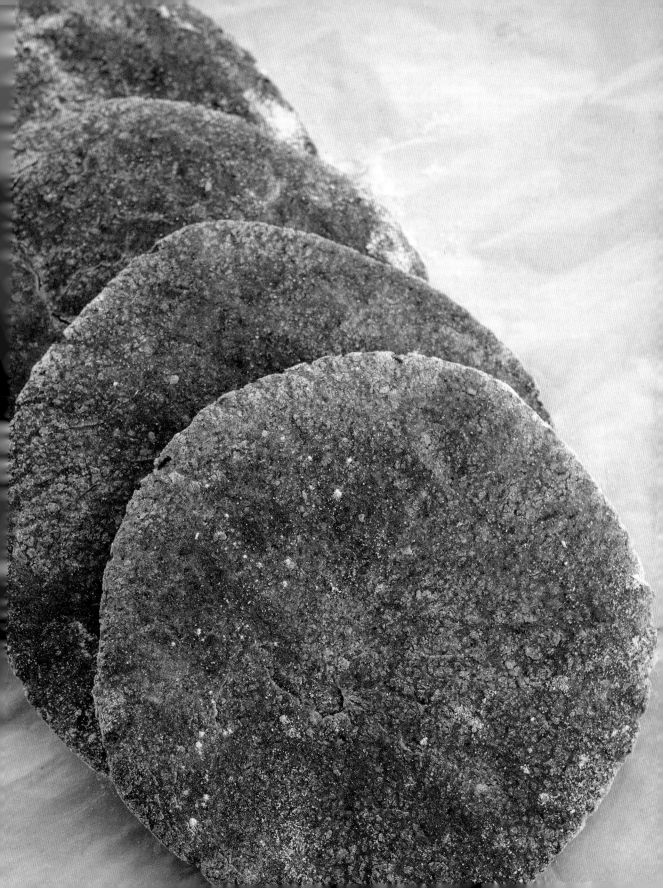

SUPER EASY FOCACCIA BREAD
(and Pizza Crust)

This must be one of my favorite recipes I've created. When I was writing this book, I was actually sad I couldn't share this recipe with you earlier. It's so easy to make, allergen friendly (nut-free and egg-free), and easy to freeze and reheat so you can make a big batch and have focaccia bread handy whenever you feel like. The texture is very close to that of normal flatbread, and it tastes like bread. Feel free to personalize it with your favorite herb combination (fresh or dried).

Preparation time:
35 minutes

Cooking time:
15 minutes

Serves:
8–10

1 cup (140 g) sorghum flour

½ cup (70 g) cassava flour

¼ cup (24 g) psyllium husk

1 teaspoon salt

1 teaspoon baking soda

1 tablespoon (2 g) chopped rosemary

Optional: dried oregano, olives, or any herbs of your choice

1 tablespoon (15 ml) apple cider vinegar

A little less than ¼ cup (50 ml) extra-virgin olive oil

1 cup (235 ml) plus ½ cup (120 ml) warm water (or less if necessary)

Sea salt flakes for topping

1. Preheat the oven to 400°F (200°C, or gas mark 6). If available, use the bread or pizza setting on your oven.

2. Combine the sorghum flour, cassava flour, psyllium husk, salt, and baking soda in a mixing bowl. Whisk so everything is combined well.

3. Add the rosemary and whatever other herbs you are using, apple cider vinegar, and olive oil and start adding the water bit by bit and mix with a spatula or wooden spoon. When the mixture becomes too hard for the spatula or spoon, start using your hands.

4. Continue to add water and knead the dough until you get a flexible, gluey dough that sticks together and is well hydrated. I usually add the first cup (235 ml) and then slowly add from the remaining ½ cup (120 ml). I never finish the entire quantity—a little less than ¼ cup (60 ml) usually remains—but it will also depend on your flour. The dough needs to stick together, and it shouldn't feel dry.

5. Split the dough into two equal parts. Use a parchment paper and roll out each one with a rolling pin until you get a round sheet about 7 inches (18 cm) in diameter. Portion with a dough cutter into eight triangles. Transfer the triangles onto a baking sheet. I remove the parchment paper for baking. I think it gets a better crust without it if you use a stainless steel pan; otherwise, keep the paper. Sprinkle with sea salt flakes.

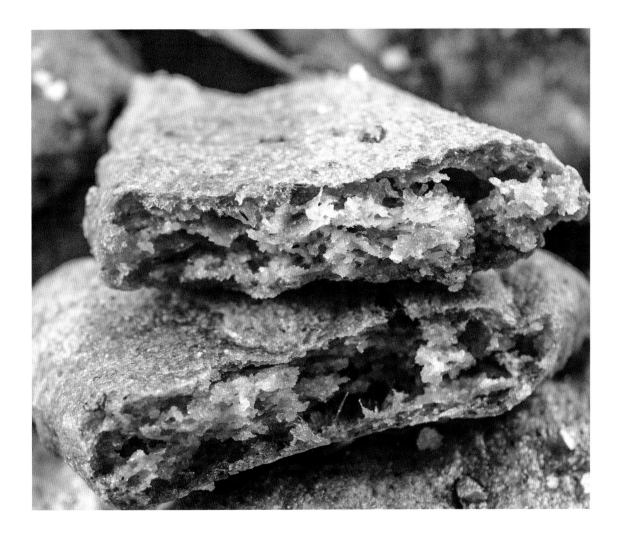

6. Bake for about 15 minutes until golden brown. Serve warm, cold, or freeze. When taking it out of the freezer, warm it in the oven, at 400°F (200°C, or gas mark 6). Time might vary slightly depending on the setting of the oven you use.

NOTE: This is my favorite way of shaping and portioning the dough after trying a few other methods. I feel it gets more evenly cooked this way, with the right proportion of crust.

HOW TO MAKE PIZZA CRUST WITH THIS DOUGH

Split the dough into four equal parts and roll them out thinner than the focaccia, about 7 inches (18 cm) in diameter. Lift the edges and poke holes with a fork on the surface. Bake for 12 minutes without toppings. You can freeze them for later use or add toppings and bake for about 8 more minutes on a pizza setting or at 400°F (200°C, or gas mark 6).

PARSNIP AND ROSEMARY CRACKERS WITH GOLDEN FLAXSEEDS

Parsnips are flavorful and easy to find. I use them in a lot of recipes: from cakes to purées to crackers. These crackers are easy to make, but they require some extra attention, as the line between perfectly crispy crackers and burnt crackers is very thin. They should be golden, not brown.

Preparation time:
35 minutes

Cooking time:
40 minutes

Makes:
About 40 crackers

About ¼ cup (47 g) golden whole flaxseeds (or ⅓ cup [37 g] ground)

¾ cup (120 g) boiled parsnip, fork-tender

About 6 tablespoons (50 ml) extra-virgin olive oil

About 6 tablespoons (50 ml) warm water (you can use the water from boiling the parsnips)

½ teaspoon salt

1 tablespoon (6 g) psyllium husk flakes

½ cup (52 g) almond flour

1 tablespoon (2 g) finely chopped fresh rosemary

3 tablespoons cassava flour (a little more if needed)

1. Preheat the oven to 350°F (180°C, or gas mark 4). Grind the flaxseeds or if already ground, use ⅓ cup (37 g). In a high-powered blender, mix the cooked parsnip, olive oil, water, and salt until creamy. Transfer the blended ingredients to a mixing bowl.

2. Add the psyllium husk, ground flaxseeds, and almond flour and combine with a spatula. Add the chopped rosemary.

3. Start adding the cassava flour and when the dough becomes thick, start kneading with your hands. You will get a nice ball of dough that holds together well.

4. Add the dough to a parchment paper sheet, spread it with your hands to get a shape as close as possible to a rectangle, and then add a sheet of parchment paper on top and roll out with a rolling pin. The thickness of the sheet should be about ⅛ inch (3 mm). The dough tends to stay thicker in the middle and thinner on the sides, so try to make it as even as possible.

5. Remove the top parchment sheet and portion the crackers with a knife, pizza cutter, or dough cutter. You can also use cookie cutters if you want to make fancier shapes, but you will have to reroll the leftover dough to reuse.

6. Poke holes with a fork into each cracker and slide the parchment paper with the dough onto a baking sheet.

7. Bake for 35 to 40 minutes. You will have to watch them and remove any crackers that are ready earlier, as the sides tend to be thinner and cook faster. After about 20 minutes, I recommend taking the baking sheet out of the oven and separating all the crackers. They'll cook more evenly. Please be careful as the line between having perfectly cooked crackers and burnt crackers is very thin (1 minute can make a huge difference). The color of the crackers should be golden, not brown. On the other hand, undercooked crackers will not get crispy. A way to check is to touch the surface of the crackers with your nails, and if it feels hard, it's done.

YUCCA ROOT AND SORGHUM PIZZA CRUST

If you are lucky to find yucca root (also called cassava), this is one of the best ways to use it. If you can't find it fresh, search the freezer section. You can also find it online or in specialty stores. This quantity will make two full-size pizzas, but you can also make four personal crusts. I make them in advance, precook, and freeze them. Whenever I want a pizza, I thaw it in the hot oven, add the sauce and toppings, and cook at 400°F (200°C, or gas mark 6) for 5 to 7 minutes. If yucca root is impossible to find, try green plantain (follow the same instructions).

Preparation time:
35 minutes

Cooking time:
10 minutes

Makes:
2 full-size crusts

1½ cups (309 g) yucca root (cassava), peeled, boiled until fork-tender, and mashed

¼ cup (60 g) coconut cream

⅛ cup (28 ml) extra-virgin olive oil

1 teaspoon salt

1 teaspoon dried oregano

2 tablespoons (12 g) psyllium husk flakes

1½ cups (210 g) sorghum flour plus 4 to 5 tablespoons (35 to 44 g) for kneading and rolling out (the amount will depend on how you measure the yucca root and how watery it is)

1. Preheat the oven to 400°F (200°C, or gas mark 6), preferably using a pizza or bread setting if available.

2. Combine the mashed (premashing is necessary just for measuring) yucca root (cassava), coconut cream, olive oil, salt, and oregano in a blender until a sticky cream forms. Transfer the mixture to a big mixing bowl.

3. Add the psyllium husk and start adding the sorghum flour bit by bit, mixing with a spatula. When a thicker dough starts to form, you can switch to mixing with your hands until you have added all the flour.

4. Knead for 5 more minutes and split the dough into two equal parts.

5. On a work surface, add a sheet of parchment paper, dust with some sorghum flour, and knead one of the dough pieces with about 2 tablespoons (18 g) of sorghum flour. When the flour is incorporated, start pressing it with your hands into a round shape. Continue to roll it out with a rolling pin until you get a round shape about 8 to 9 inches (20 to 23 cm) in diameter.

6. Transfer the dough to a baking sheet by sliding the paper onto the tray. Poke holes with a fork on the surface of the pizza crust.

7. Repeat with the second crust, if making two pizzas. If not, you can make the second crust later, prebake, and freeze.

8. Bake for about 10 minutes without any toppings. You need to make sure that the crust is completely cooked (no longer soft) before you add the toppings. Remove it from the oven and place it on a cooling rack. Cooking time may vary slightly depending on the oven.

9. If making a pizza immediately, take the baked crust, add the sauce and the toppings, and bake for about 5 to 7 more minutes or until the crust is crispy on the edges and the toppings are done.

10. If you don't make the pizza immediately, let the pizza crust cool down completely and freeze for later use. Make sure you add parchment paper in between each crust so they don't stick to each other.

EASY CASSAVA FLOUR TORTILLAS

These are more than a staple in our house. Everyone loves them, even those who would usually eat normal bread. They are pliable, easy to make, and only require four ingredients, if you count water and salt. Make a big batch in advance and freeze them, stacking them with parchment paper in between. Take out of the freezer and warm on a pan or in the oven. Depending on how long you warm them for, they'll be soft and pliable, or they can become crispy to make perfect tostadas or tortilla chips. A tortilla press can come in handy and will speed up the process.

Preparation time:
30 minutes

Cooking time:
50 minutes

Makes:
8–10 tortillas (8 inches [20 cm])

1½ cups (200 g) plus 1 tablespoon (9 g) super fine cassava flour

1 teaspoon salt

3 tablespoons (45 ml) extra-virgin olive oil

1½ cups (355 ml) warm water

1. Add the flour, salt, and olive oil to a big mixing bowl. Combine with a spatula.

2. Start adding water and continue to stir so the ingredients come together. When it gets too solid, start kneading with your hands and continue to add water, bit by bit.

3. The kneading part is very important and will make all the difference. Continue to knead (like you would knead normal bread) and add water. The whole process can take about 10 minutes. The dough will be hydrated and elastic but should not get sticky. The moment it gets sticky, there is too much water, which can easily be fixed by dusting it with a little bit of flour.

4. Shape the dough into a ball and portion it into eight equal parts. Shape them into small balls.

5. Heat a cast-iron pan on the stove.

6. Take one ball, flatten it out on a sheet of parchment paper, add another parchment paper on top, and roll it out into a round shape with a rolling pin. If you feel it is a little sticky, dust the surface with a tiny bit of cassava flour.

7. Peel the top paper off. You can leave the tortilla as it is, or if you want a perfect round shape, you can place a soup bowl on top and trim around the edges. Keep the leftovers. You will have enough dough to make two more tortillas at the end. Irregular shapes are also nice if you don't want to bother with this extra step.

8. The tortillas should come off the paper easily, only using your hands or a spatula. If not, another way to put it in the pan is to take the paper with the

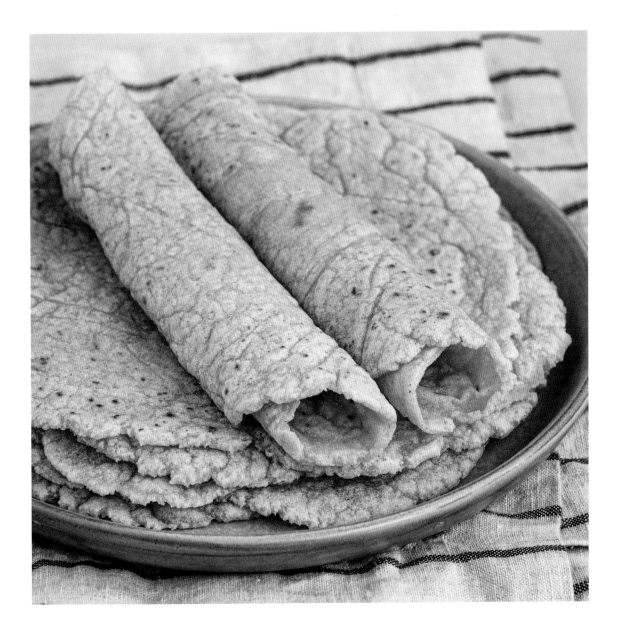

tortilla on top and flip it onto the pan. Make sure the pan is hot when you put the tortilla on. With practice, you will figure out what the best strategy is for you.

9. Cook the tortillas for about 2 to 3 minutes on one side until brown blisters form. Then, flip and cook for 2 to 3 more minutes. When you flip, it should make pockets, but if it doesn't, don't worry—they'll be just as good.

10. Once a tortilla is done, put it on a plate, without covering it (I find they get too soft if covered). Continue to add warm ones on top. They'll provide just enough moisture to the other ones to keep them all soft until you finish. I roll out tortillas while I wait for the previous ones to cook. If you have a tortilla press, it will go a little faster.

SORGHUM MORNING BREAD ROLLS

I learned how to make morning bread rolls (*rundstykker* in Danish) from my Danish mother-in-law many years ago. They were made with graham flour. While spending one of the past summers in Denmark, where bread is everything, I felt like creating a lectin-free version of rundstykker, and this is the result. I make a big batch in advance, freeze them, and then heat them up in a hot oven right before eating. Having these warm buns to spread butter and a homemade jam on is everything.

Preparation time:
30 minutes

Cooking time:
50 minutes–1 hour

Makes:
12 morning bread rolls

DRY INGREDIENTS:

2 cups (280 g) sorghum flour

½ cup (56 g) ground flaxseeds

½ cup (60 g) tigernut flour

½ cup (52 g) almond flour

¼ cup (24 g) psyllium husk

1½ teaspoons salt

WET INGREDIENTS:

¾ cup (175 ml) full-fat coconut milk

3 tablespoons (45 ml) fresh lemon juice

1 cup (235 ml) warm water

2 tablespoons (28 ml) extra-virgin olive oil

¼ cup (36 g) sesame seeds

1. Preheat the oven to 400°F (200°C, or gas mark 6) and prepare a baking sheet (in my experience, there is no need for greasing or for parchment paper).

2. Mix the coconut milk with the lemon juice and let it sit for about 10 to 15 minutes.

3. Mix the dry ingredients in a big bowl.

4. Add the coconut milk and lemon juice mixture, water, and olive oil. Gently knead the dough and form a ball.

5. Portion the ball in 12 equal parts. Don't overshape or press them down too much, as they will get denser. Repeat with all the dough and when done, dip the top side of each roll in the sesame seeds.

6. Arrange all the bread rolls on the baking sheet and bake for about 1 hour, keeping an eye on them, as they might be ready earlier. I like to get a crust, so I prefer to cook them longer.

7. I like to make a double batch and freeze. You can warm them up in the preheated oven (400°F [200°C, or gas mark 6]), straight from the freezer, for about 10 minutes.

SPICY KETO CRACKERS WITH DUKKAH

These crackers go with everything, add a little kick to a meal, are the perfect snack on the go, and keep you satiated. I wanted to offer a keto version to those of you who follow diets lower in carbohydrates. These crackers are really easy to make, even for a beginner, and are not boring. The spice mix is very easy to make. I always have a jar in the refrigerator. For this recipe, you will just have to grind it finer, using a coffee grinder or a nutribullet with a milling blade.

Preparation time:
20 minutes

Cooking time:
20 minutes

Makes:
About 60 crackers

½ cup (56 g) finely ground flaxseed meal (for a lighter taste and color, use golden flaxseed)

⅓ cup (43 g) Dukkah Spice and Nut Mix (page 28)

1 cup (104 g) almond flour (pressed down or packed)

Spices: about ½–1 teaspoon each: dried rosemary, thyme, oregano, cumin, sumac, and freshly ground pepper

⅔ teaspoon pink Himalayan salt

1 tablespoon (15 ml) extra-virgin olive oil

8 tablespoons (120 ml) water

1. Heat the oven to 350°F (180°C, or gas mark 4) and prepare a large baking sheet.

2. The best way to use flaxseeds is to grind them yourself with a coffee grinder or a nutribullet with a milling blade. Store-bought flaxseed meal can be used, but make sure it is fresh and not rancid (fishy smelling). The next step is to grind the Dukkah Spice and Nut Mix finer. The usual dukkah is a bit coarse, so before using it in this recipe, you need to finely grind it. Mix the almond flour with the ground flaxseed, dukkah, spices, and salt. Add the olive oil.

3. Start adding the water tablespoon by tablespoon and mix. It will get moist and stick together. Form a ball and let it rest for 5 minutes.

4. Place the dough on a piece of parchment paper, press a little with your hands to get a rectangle shape, cover with another sheet of parchment paper, and roll out gently with a rolling pin, trying to make as much of a rectangular shape as possible, until the dough has the thickness of a cracker (about ⅛ inch [3 mm]).

5. Gently remove the top paper and slide the bottom paper with the dough on top of the sheet pan. Portion with a pizza cutter or knife in squares or rectangles and poke holes with a fork (this will make them look like crackers and will also help them cook more evenly).

6. Bake for about 20 minutes, turn the heat off, and leave them in the oven for another 5 minutes. Like any cracker, it needs to be watched carefully, so don't rely on the timer. After 12 minutes, keep an eye on them, and if you see they start getting crispy or burning, turn the heat off. Sometimes, the sides are thinner so they will get cooked faster. If you see that, you can take those crackers out first.

7. They can be stored in the fridge in an airtight glass jar for a few days. They will stay crispy.

FAUX "CORN BREAD" WITH MILLET AND WALNUTS

A lectin-free makeover of the much-loved staple, corn bread, this is as good if not even better. Before corn was introduced to Europe, bread and polenta were made of millet, so replacing corn with millet is not such a novelty. Ground millet has a similar texture to corn flour and can easily be made at home with a food processor or blender and a milling blade (I use a nutribullet, but a coffee or spice grinder would work too). Don't use store-bought millet flour; the texture is too fine for this bread. Eat warm with butter and local or raw honey or serve it as a side to savory dishes.

Preparation time:
15 minutes

Cooking time:
30 minutes

Serves:
10

DRY INGREDIENTS:

1½ cups (300 g) millet, coarsely ground

1 cup (100 g) walnuts, ground

¼ cup (30 g) tapioca flour

¼ cup (35 g) cassava flour

½ teaspoon baking powder

½ teaspoon baking soda

⅛ teaspoon salt

WET INGREDIENTS:

1 cup (240 g) coconut cream

2–3 tablespoons (28 to 45 ml) fresh lemon juice

1 pastured egg

¼ cup (60 ml) extra-virgin olive oil

1 tablespoon (20 g) local or raw honey

1 teaspoon pure vanilla extract

Zest of 1 organic lemon

1. Mix the coconut cream with the lemon juice and set it aside for 10 to 15 minutes to slightly curdle.

2. Preheat the oven to 350°F (180°C, or gas mark 4).

3. Prepare one baking dish. I used a Pyrex, approximately 7 x 11 inches (18 x 28 cm), with low walls (it helps with release). If you can, line the baking dish with parchment paper.

4. Grind the millet in a food processor (I use my nutribullet with the milling blade) until it resembles corn flour (not too coarse, not too fine).

5. Grind the walnuts in the same processor. It doesn't matter if it's not uniform and there are some bigger pieces left; they will add to the texture.

6. Combine all the dry ingredients in a big bowl.

7. Combine all the wet ingredients in a smaller bowl, mixing with a whisk just until they all get combined. There's no need to overmix.

8. Add the wet ingredients to the dry, combine well with a spatula, and if you feel like the batter is too dry, add a little bit of water.

9. Transfer the batter to the baking dish, level with the spatula, and bake for about 30 minutes until golden brown on top and a toothpick comes out clean.

10. Store in an airtight container in a cool place or in the fridge for up to 2 days. It can also be frozen.

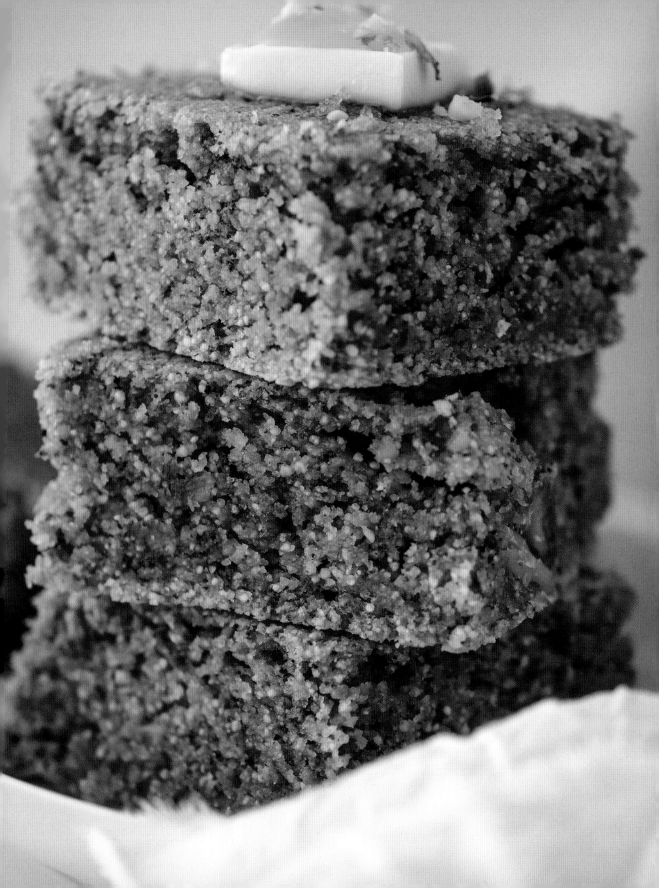

GREEN GNOCCHI WITH ARUGULA AND CASSAVA FLOUR

Homemade gnocchi are a great meal plan item you can prepare in advance, freeze, and use whenever you need to put together an easy but delicious weeknight meal. Don't get discouraged by the 1½ hours of preparation. During this time, you will make 80 gnocchi, which is about 8 servings. They are easy to cook straight from the freezer. Just sauté them with onion and garlic, maybe some seafood or sausage, and add cream or a nut milk for a creamy consistency.

Preparation time:
1 hour
30 minutes

Cooking time:
50 minutes

Makes:
80 gnocchi

FOR THE GREEN PURÉE:

2½ cups (50 g) arugula, packed (or use other greens)

2 spring onions

2 spring garlic (green garlic) or 3 garlic cloves, minced

4 tablespoons (60 ml) extra-virgin olive oil

¼ cup (60 ml) water

1 teaspoon salt

FOR THE DOUGH:

2 pastured eggs

1¼ cups (285 ml) hemp milk, homemade (page 33) or store-bought

1½ cups (210 g) cassava flour, divided into 1 cup (140 g) and ½ cup (70 g)

2 tablespoons (28 ml) sparkling water

Zest of 1 organic lemon

1. Fill a big pot with water, about ⅔ full, and start heating the water.

2. Make the green purée: Blend all the ingredients until liquid and smooth.

3. Make the dough: In a food processor, add the eggs, hemp milk, 1 cup (140 g) cassava flour, sparkling water, and lemon zest. Process until it forms a soft dough.

4. Add the green purée and pulse a few times until combined. In case your food processor is not big enough, you can also combine the soft dough and the green purée in a mixing bowl.

5. Start adding the remaining ½ cup (70 g) of cassava flour gradually and mix with a spatula. When it becomes too thick, start kneading with your hands. You will get a homogenous, elastic dough, resembling Play-Doh consistency.

6. Shape it into a big ball and then split it into four equal parts. From each part, you will roll two logs, about the thickness of your thumb. Each log will be about 10 inches (25 cm) long. You will cut 10 gnocchi from each log.

7. You can cook the gnocchi as they are, but if you have some extra time and don't want to skip the fun part, use a gnocchi ridger to shape them. If not, a fork will work as well. Place the fork with the tips of the tines on the surface and gently roll each gnocchi down the tines.

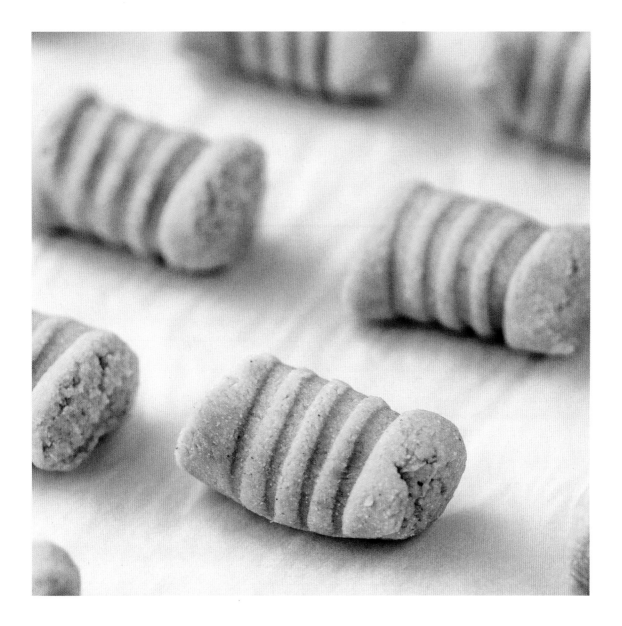

8. By this time, the water should be boiling. Turn the heat to low and add the first batch of gnocchi (20 gnocchi total), with the help of a slotted spoon. You can start preparing the second batch while the first one cooks.

9. After about 4 minutes, the gnocchi will start to float. Take them out with a slotted spoon and put them on a dry surface or plate. Repeat with the next three batches.

10. When they are all ready, you can prepare them or let them cool completely, add them to a container separating each layer with parchment paper, and freeze them (add paper on the bottom and on top too).

11. To prepare them, you can sauté them with the rest of your chosen ingredients straight from the freezer.

EVERYDAY, NUTRITIOUS, AND TASTY LITTLE BREADS

These *little breads* are so flavorful and satisfying. My dad said they taste like meatballs. I wanted to create something that delivers more than just a bread replacement. They are nutrient dense, delicious, and can be used in so many different combinations. I absolutely love them in the summer with peeled and deseeded tomatoes from the garden, extra-virgin olive oil, olives, oregano, and a little bit of mozzarella.

Preparation time:
30 minutes

Cooking time:
25 minutes

Makes:
8 little breads

DRY INGREDIENTS:

3 tablespoons (20 g) flaxseed meal

1 tablespoon (9 g) arrowroot powder

2 tablespoons (12 g) psyllium husk

1 cup (130 g) cassava flour, plus more if necessary for kneading

2½ tablespoons (20 g) tigernut flour

2 tablespoons (19 g) hemp seeds

¼ cup (25 g) almond flour

1 teaspoon baking powder

1 tablespoon (6 g) black cumin seeds (Nigella sativa)

½ tablespoon herbs de Provence

1 teaspoon dried oregano

1 teaspoon salt

WET INGREDIENTS:

1 small onion, chopped

2–3 garlic cloves

½ cup (160 g) sweet potato purée (boiled or baked)

1 teaspoon apple cider vinegar

¼ cup (60 ml) full-fat coconut milk

¼ cup (60 ml) water

5 tablespoons (75 ml) extra-virgin olive oil

1. Preheat the oven to 400°F (200°C, or gas mark 6) and prepare a baking sheet with parchment paper. Prepare another parchment sheet and a rolling pin.

2. Combine all the dry ingredients in a big mixing bowl.

3. Add all the wet ingredients to a blender and combine until creamy and smooth.

4. Add the wet ingredients to the dry ingredients in the mixing bowl and combine with a spatula, then with your hands, until you form a nice ball of dough. If you feel like the dough is too wet, you can sprinkle more cassava flour and knead. If it is too dry, wet your hands and knead until the dough gets more hydrated.

5. Split the dough in eight equal balls and flatten them with your hands or with the help of a rolling pin. From my experience, there is no need for a top sheet of parchment paper, but just in case you feel the dough will stick to the rolling pin, you can do that. Roll them about ¼ inch (6 mm) thick.

6. Transfer the little breads onto the baking sheet and bake for about 25 minutes. I like when the crust gets a little hard. There is nothing in the dough (like eggs) that needs to cook in order to be safe to eat, so you can vary the timing to suit your taste.

7. You can freeze them and reheat in the oven.

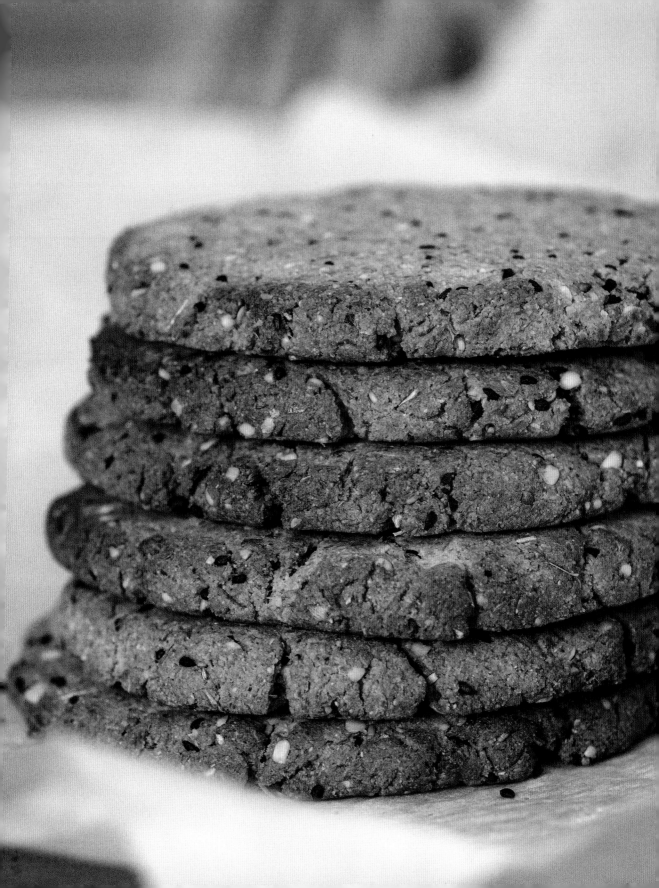

EASY KETO PIE CRUST, WITHOUT EGGS

For a gluten-free dough, this keto-friendly dough is sturdy and easy to work with. I use it to make sweet potato pie and apple or cherry galette, or you can use it with savory fillings or to make quiche.

Preparation time:
20 minutes

Cooking time:
About 30–35 minutes, depending on pie filling

Makes:
One 8-inch (20 cm) pie crust

1 cup (104 g) almond flour, pressed down

½ cup (56 g) coconut flour

¼ cup (36 g) arrowroot flour

Pinch of salt

6 tablespoons (80 g) cold grass-fed butter, cubed

¼ cup (60 ml) ice-cold water plus 1–2 tablespoons (15 to 28 ml)

1 small cube grass-fed butter, for greasing the pie dish

1. Add all the dry ingredients to a food processor and pulse until combined.

2. Add the butter and pulse a few times until you see a grainy consistency.

3. With the food processor running on low, add the ice-cold water. Start with ¼ cup (60 ml) and add 1 or 2 extra tablespoons (15 to 28 ml) until you get a doughy consistency. You don't want the dough to be too hydrated, but not too dry either.

4. Take the dough out, shape into a ball, wrap in plastic, and store in the fridge for about an hour.

5. Preheat the oven to 350°F (180°C, or gas mark 4).

6. Prepare a pie dish by greasing it with butter.

7. Take the dough out of the fridge, put on top of a parchment paper sheet, and gently flatten it with your hands. Add another parchment sheet on top and gently roll the dough out with a rolling pin until you get a diameter of about 10 inches (25 cm). If edges start to crack, delicately push them back in, cover with the paper, and gently roll around the edges.

8. Peel the top paper off and with the help of the bottom paper, carefully flip the dough on top of the pic dish. This dough should be pretty sturdy and not crack, but if it does, it's easy to stick back together. Fit it into the dish and remove the excess dough, add the filling, and bake.

9. You can also use this dough to make galette- or crostata-style pies.

KETO AND VEGAN LOAF BREAD

They say necessity teaches us. I had to come up with a keto bread for my dad when he needed to remove most carbs from his diet. Making keto bread using many eggs is quite easy, but a keto bread that is also vegan is quite the challenge. I'm sharing this recipe because all of my bread-loving family likes it, and it's so easy to make. It holds the shape very well and while it looks dense, it has a light bite. It's also a moist bread that will not dry out easily. I like to slice it and freeze it and thaw it naturally or using a toaster or a sandwich maker. The Nigella sativa seeds, also known as black cumin seeds, give this bread a special flavor, but if you don't like this taste, you can leave them out. Basil seeds can be skipped if you can't find them, and the xanthan gum can be skipped, although it adds a little bit of texture.

Preparation time:
25 minutes

Cooking time:
1 hour

Makes:
1 loaf bread

DRY INGREDIENTS:

1 cup (104 g) almond flour, packed

½ cup (60 g) tigernut flour

⅓ cup (37 g) coconut flour

3 tablespoons (21 g) hazelnut flour

4 tablespoons (24 g) psyllium husk flakes

4 tablespoons (28 g) ground flaxseeds

1 teaspoon salt

2 teaspoons baking powder

1 teaspoon xanthan gum

1 tablespoon (13 g) basil seeds

1 tablespoon (6 g) black cumin seeds (Nigella sativa)

2 tablespoons (19 g) hemp seeds

2 tablespoons (32 g) nut butter or (30 g) tahini

WET INGREDIENTS:

1 tablespoon (15 ml) extra-virgin olive oil

1 tablespoon (15 ml) apple cider vinegar

1 cup (235 ml) plus 2 tablespoons (28 ml) hot water

1. Line a small loaf pan with parchment paper (a 3-cup [700 ml] volume loaf pan, measured ⅔ full, or two mini loaf pans).

2. Mix all the dry ingredients in a large bowl.

3. Add the olive oil and apple cider vinegar and start adding the hot water and mix.

4. Knead gently until you get a dough. Let it rest for 5 minutes and shape it into a log the size of your loaf pan.

5. Bake for 1 hour at 375°F (190°C, or gas mark 5) until it forms a golden brown crust. If you are unsure about doneness, you can use the toothpick test. Remove from the pan and let it cool completely before slicing. It will last for a few days in the fridge, or it can be frozen. It can also be toasted before serving.

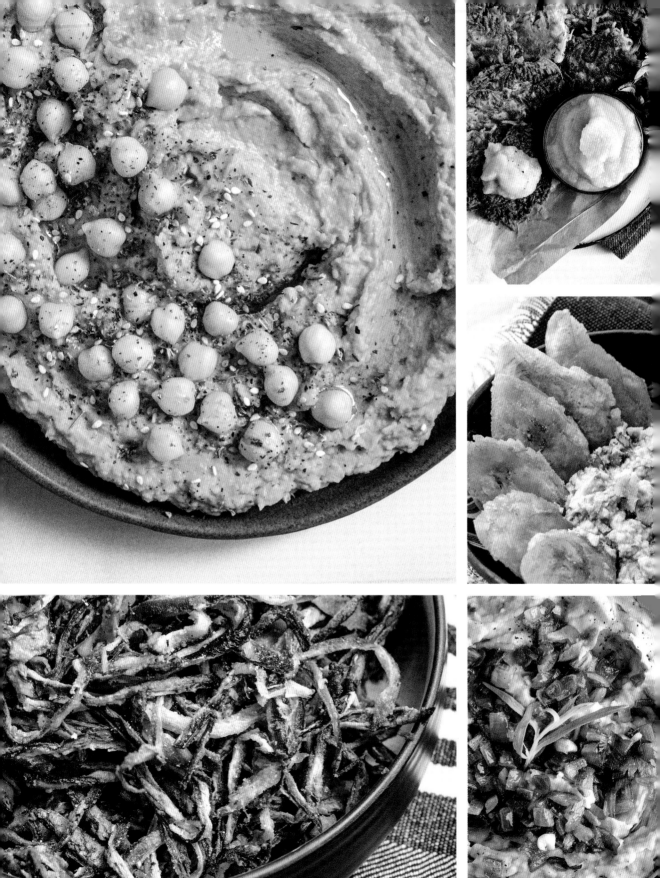

4

Appetizers and Small Bites

Clockwise from top left: Chickpea and Roasted Pepper Hummus with Zaatar Spice (page 74); Parsnip and Sweet Potato Fritters (Latkes) with Homemade Apple Sauce (page 76); Tostones and Guacamole (page 72); White Bean Cream with Red Onion and Fennel (page 77); Oven-Baked Crispy Onions (page 73)

TOSTONES AND GUACAMOLE

This is the perfect appetizer, snack, or breakfast, and why not make it a full meal? To me, tostones and guacamole can be anything. Add an egg to the combo, and you have a meal that'll keep you full for the day. Make it part of a tapas menu and impress your guests.

Preparation time:
30 minutes

Cooking time:
25 minutes

Serves:
2

FOR THE TOSTONES:

1 green plantain

A generous layer of extra-virgin olive oil or avocado oil

Salt

FOR THE GUACAMOLE:

1 ripe avocado

1 tablespoon (15 ml) extra-virgin olive oil

1 tablespoon (10 g) finely chopped red onion

½ lime

Salt and freshly ground pepper to taste

1 small handful of chopped cilantro

Optional: a few drops of Tabasco Red Pepper Sauce

1. To make the guacamole: Smash the avocado in a small bowl with a fork. Add the rest of the ingredients, gently mix, cover, and store in the fridge until the tostones are ready.

2. To make the tostones: Peel the plantain. (See sidebar for details on how to peel the plantain.) Slice the plantain at an angle, about 1 inch (2.5 cm) thick.

3. In a big frying pan, add olive oil or avocado oil, enough to generously cover the pan, but not too much. They will be shallow frying, and we don't want to waste too much oil. The heat used is low to medium.

4. When the oil is hot, add the slices to the pan and fry on one side for about 4 minutes. Flip them and fry again for another 4 minutes on the second side.

5. Remove them to a cutting board and smash each chunk with the bottom of a glass or jar, applying gentle pressure so they don't break. Carefully remove from the bottom of the glass if they get stuck. Put them back into the pan and fry again on low heat for about 2 to 3 minutes on each side.

6. Remove from the pan and generously season with salt. Serve with the guacamole.

HOW TO PEEL A GREEN PLANTAIN

1. Wash the green plantain with warm or hot water and let the water run on it for a couple of minutes.

2. Pat dry and cut both ends of the plantain.

3. With a good paring knife, slit along the length of the plantain in three or four places.

4. Slide the knife under the edge of the peel and start loosening it bit by bit, peeling to the side, not lengthwise like a normal banana.

5. Be careful not to cut deeper than the skin, especially if you make tostones or chips.

OVEN BAKED CRISPY ONIONS

These are a great addition to vegetable bowls, open sandwiches, burgers, dipping sauces, and even soups.

Preparation time:
10 minutes

Cooking time:
35 minutes

Serves:
2–4

1 medium red onion

1 pastured egg

1 tablespoon (15 ml) extra-virgin olive oil

⅛ teaspoon salt

⅛ teaspoon freshly ground pepper

2 tablespoons (18 g) cassava flour

1. Preheat the oven to 400°F (200°C, or gas mark 6).

2. Cut the onion in half and then slice each half as finely as you can, making sure the slices are not attached to each other.

3. Beat the egg in a large bowl, add the olive oil, salt, and pepper, and combine. Then, add the onions to the bowl and with your hands, mix the onion and the egg so the onion slices get coated with the egg.

4. Remove the onion slices from the bowl and spread on a large stainless steel baking sheet, so there is as little overlap as possible.

5. Add 1 tablespoon (9 g) of the flour to a sieve and sift it all over the onion slices. Mix them around the sheet with two forks and repeat with the second tablespoon (9 g) of flour. Mix again with the forks and spread the onion slices on the baking sheet.

6. Bake for about 20 minutes, stir again with tongs or forks, and bake for 15 more minutes or until they are crispy. Remove from the oven and let them cool on the baking sheet.

7. Serve warm or cold.

8. You can store leftovers in a glass container in the fridge for 2 to 3 days. They won't stay super crispy, but you can pop them in the oven again and they'll crisp up.

CHICKPEA AND ROASTED PEPPER HUMMUS WITH ZAATAR SPICE

This hummus is a crowd pleaser. You can pressure cook the chickpeas, or you can use canned chickpeas, preferably organic and BPA-free. Roasted peppers that are peeled and deseeded can be found in stores, or you can easily roast them in the oven. Serve with raw vegetable sticks or Parsnip and Rosemary Crackers with Golden Flaxsees (page 56).

Preparation time:
15 minutes

Serves:
4–6

2 cups (328 g) pressure cooked chickpeas (or use canned chickpeas, drained and rinsed)

½ cup (90 g) roasted peppers, chopped

3 tablespoons (45 ml) extra-virgin olive oil

1 tablespoon (15 g) tahini

½–1 teaspoon salt to your taste

½ teaspoon ground cumin

⅛–¼ teaspoon freshly ground pepper

1 small garlic clove, minced

4 tablespoons (60 ml) cold water

2 tablespoons (28 ml) fresh lemon juice

FOR GARNISHING:

2 teaspoons zaatar mix

1 tablespoon (15 ml) extra-virgin olive oil

Whole chickpeas

Optional: sea salt flakes

1. Add all the ingredients to a blender or food processor, starting with just ½ teaspoon salt, and process until creamy. If you use a food processor, it will be more chunky. If you use a blender, it will be more smooth and creamy. Taste and adjust the salt or any other spices if necessary.

2. Plate and garnish with zaatar spice mix, extra-virgin olive oil, and whole chickpeas. I like to finish with some sea salt flakes.

3. Store in the fridge in a glass container for 2 to 3 days.

HOW TO PRESSURE COOK CHICKPEAS

Soak them overnight, changing the water several times. Pressure cook for 25 minutes. For more flavor, you can add fresh rosemary, yellow onion, and carrots to the water.

HOW TO ROAST PEPPERS IN THE OVEN

Wash and dry the peppers and roast them at 400°F (200°C, or gas mark 6) for about 30 minutes or until they form blisters on all sides. Add them to a bowl, sprinkle with salt, and cover for about 10 minutes. They'll soften and the peel will come off easily.

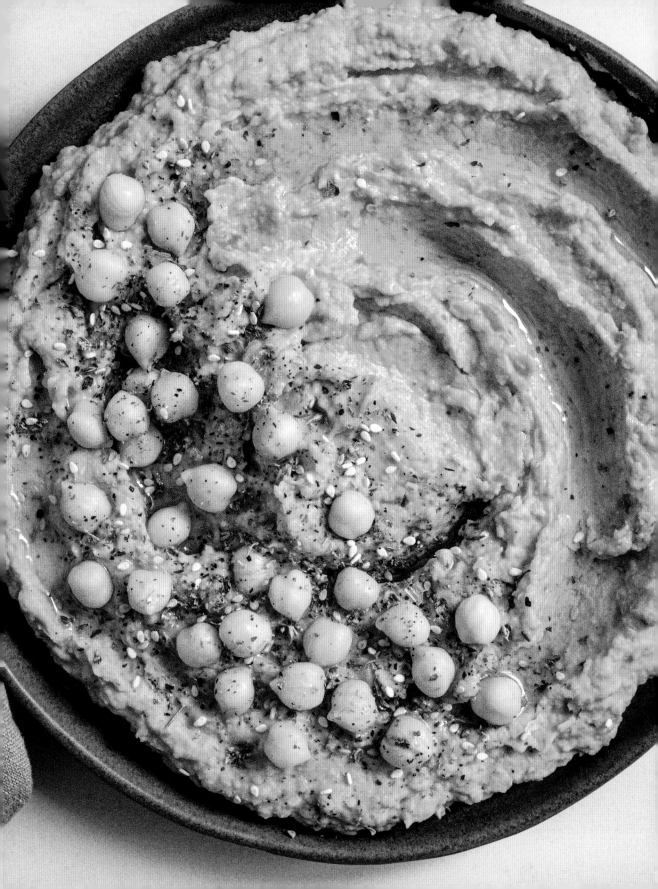

PARSNIP AND SWEET POTATO FRITTERS (LATKES) WITH HOMEMADE APPLESAUCE

A nightshade-free version of the famous *latkes*, this recipe was created to provide a delicious alternative to those who can't have white potatoes. Even if latkes are not part of your holiday tradition, they are easy to make and so tasty, anyone would love them.

Preparation time:
20 minutes

Cooking time:
25 minutes

Serves:
4–6

FOR THE APPLESAUCE:

3 medium Fuji apples, peeled, cored, and cubed

¼ cup (60 ml) filtered water

FOR THE SWEET POTATO FRITTERS:

1 medium Japanese sweet potato (purple skin, white flesh), peeled and grated

1 big parsnip, rubbed clean and grated

1 pastured egg, beaten (or use an egg replacement)

2 tablespoons (18 g) cassava flour

3 tablespoons (21 g) almond flour

2 teaspoons sea salt

Freshly ground pepper

¼ teaspoon allspice

Optional: 1 small onion, grated

Extra-virgin olive oil or avocado oil for shallow frying

Optional: organic sour cream

1. To make the applesauce: Add the cubed apples to a pot and start warming up on the stove on low-to-medium heat. After about 10 minutes, add ¼ cup (60 ml) water and simmer on low-to-medium heat for another 20 minutes or until the apples are very soft. Add to a blender and blend until smooth. Cool and store in a glass jar in the fridge until the fritters are ready to serve.

2. To make the fritters: Mix the grated sweet potatoes and parsnip, put them into a cheesecloth, and try to squeeze as much liquid as possible (add the onions too if using). Add the veggies to a bowl and add the rest of the ingredients. Mix well until all the ingredients are combined. You can add more flour if you feel the mixture is too watery (especially if you choose to add onion).

3. Heat a large frying pan on medium heat and generously cover with your choice of oil (avocado or olive oil). When hot, start spooning heaping tablespoons (15 ml) of the mix into the pan and gently flatten out. Let them cook undisturbed until they get golden brown on one side and then flip using a spatula. Depending on how big your pan is, you probably need to make them in two batches. Make sure you let them crisp up and get brown on each side before you take them out and place on a paper towel.

4. You can keep them warm in the oven or even serve them cold. Serve the fritters with the applesauce or with organic sour cream.

WHITE BEAN CREAM WITH RED ONION AND FENNEL

In Romania, chickpeas are not very popular, but we have our own hummus. It's made of creamy white beans, lots of garlic, and onions fried in sunflower oil all mixed with tomato sauce. That's a no for me, so I made my own healthier version. I left the tomato sauce out, used a good quality extra-virgin olive oil, pressure cooked the beans, added some more flavors and spices, and created a delicious, healthy, and nutritious creamy dip. I like to serve it with raw vegetable sticks, such as carrots, celery, kohlrabi, and radishes. It makes for a great office lunch or picnic snack.

Preparation time:
30 minutes

Serves:
6

2 big red onions, finely chopped

½ fennel bulb, finely chopped

2 tablespoons (28 ml) extra-virgin olive oil

½ teaspoon ground cumin

½ teaspoon paprika

⅛ teaspoon nutmeg

4 cups (716 g) soaked and pressure cooked white beans (soak overnight and pressure cook for 30 minutes, discarding the water)

1–2 garlic cloves, minced

½ teaspoon salt

Freshly ground pepper

4–5 tablespoons (60 to 75 ml) extra-virgin olive oil

A squeeze of lime

More salt and freshly ground pepper to taste

1. Sauté the onion and fennel with the olive oil in a skillet on low heat until soft and fragrant, about 10 to 15 minutes. If you feel it needs some extra moisture and to avoid sticking to the pan, you can add 1 to 2 tablespoons (15 to 28 ml) of water.

2. When the onions and fennel are almost done, add the cumin, paprika, and nutmeg, mix well, and take off the heat.

3. Add the beans, ¾ of the onion mixture, and the rest of the ingredients to a food processor and combine until creamy or to your desired consistency.

4. Taste and season if necessary. Plate and top with ¼ of the onion and fennel mixture.

5. Serve as a dip with raw vegetable sticks, crackers, or as a creamy side dish.

GREEN PLANTAIN CHIPS

This is one of my favorite crunchy snacks ever! When I temporarily moved back to my small hometown in Romania, I was ready to give up green plantain chips. But, to my surprise, I did find green plantains in a local supermarket. While they are easy to personalize, my favorite way to make them is with coconut oil and salt. You can add any spices you want and create a sweet, savory, or spicy profile.

Preparation time:
10 minutes

Cooking time:
20 minutes

Serves:
4

1 green plantain

2 tablespoons (28 g) coconut oil (preferably solid)

Salt to taste

1. Preheat the oven to 350°F (180°C, or gas mark 4).

2. Peel the plantain and slice it with a mandolin, at a slight angle. The thickness should be about $\frac{1}{16}$ inch (2 mm).

3. Place the slices on a large baking tray, add the solid coconut oil, and generously coat each slice with the coconut oil (using your hands). Add more oil if necessary. Arrange them on the tray, next to each other, without overlapping.

4. Bake for about 20 minutes or until golden brown and crispy. Sprinkle with salt.

5. You can eat immediately or store on the counter in an airtight container for 1 to 2 days.

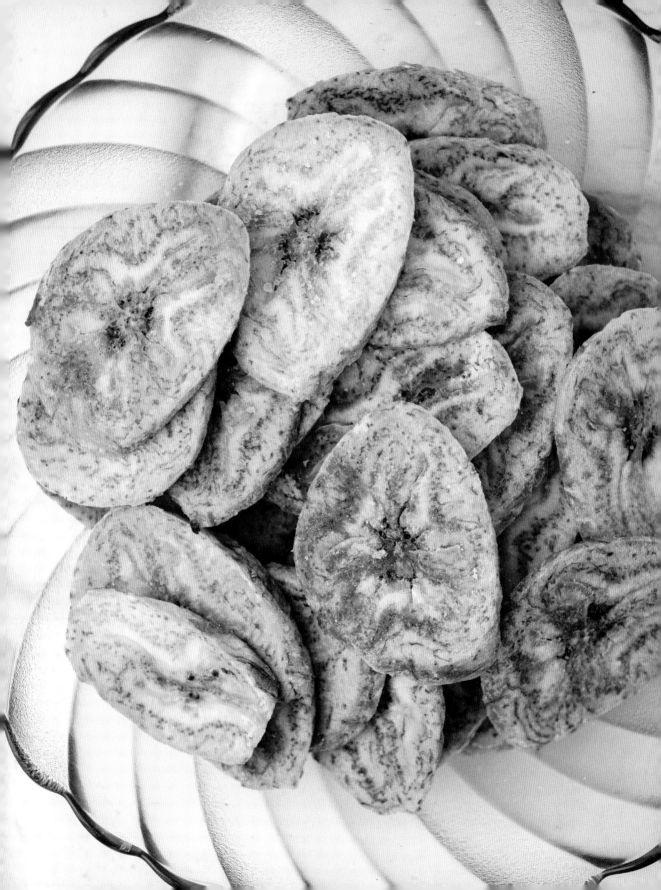

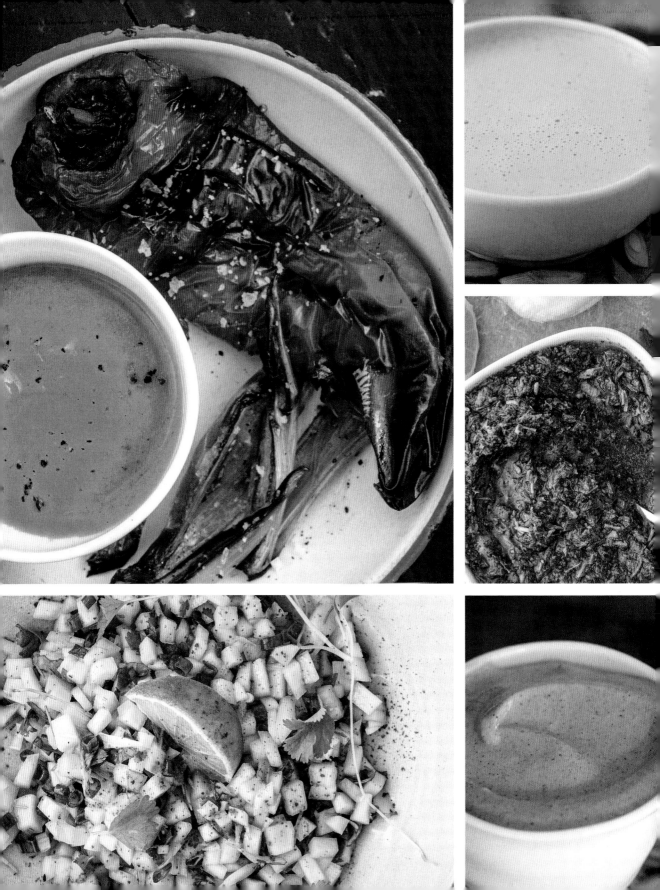

5

Sauces and Dressings

Clockwise from top left: Roasted Red Pepper Vinaigrette (page 85); Green Garlic Sauce (page 91);
Gremolata Sauce with Mint (page 82); No-Peanuts Satay Sauce (page 83); Green Mango Salsa (page 89)

GREMOLATA SAUCE WITH MINT

Gremolata is the name of an Italian chunky mix of fresh parsley, lemon zest, and garlic. I started with the traditional Italian condiment formula and transformed it into a multipurpose, delicious sauce: gremolata sauce with mint. Use it fresh. It will brighten up any kind of meat, eggs, or roasted vegetables, or use it as a marinade or salad dressing.

Preparation time:

20 minutes

Serves:

6

2½ cups (150 g) chopped parsley (washed and dried)

1 handful of fresh mint leaves (washed and dried)

1 spring garlic (green garlic), chopped, or 2 garlic cloves, grated

½ cup (120 ml) extra-virgin olive oil

Zest of 2 organic lemons (grated)

Juice of ½ lemon or to taste

¼ teaspoon salt or to taste

⅛ teaspoon freshly ground pepper

1. Add the parsley, mint, and garlic to a food processor (not a blender). Pulse until everything is chopped. It's okay to have a rougher texture. That's how gremolata should be. Start adding the olive oil and continue to mix until you added all the oil.

2. Add the lemon zest, lemon juice, and the spices and mix.

3. Serve or store in a glass jar in the fridge for a few days.

NO-PEANUTS SATAY SAUCE

It took me years to create a version of satay sauce that I was happy with. And finally, it happened. This lectin-free satay sauce is creamy, sticky, rich, and the perfect accompaniment to lectin-free Baked Chicken Satay (page 128). But feel free to pair it with other dishes. It works well with stir-fries, cabbage, and beef and makes for a perfect creamy dressing for a chicken salad. For more depth of flavor, I recommend roasted or toasted tahini, which means it was made with toasted sesame seeds (as opposed to raw tahini).

Preparation time:
30 minutes

Cooking time:
10 minutes

Makes:
1 cup (256 g)

1 shallot, finely chopped

1 garlic clove, smashed and chopped

3 heaping tablespoons (45 g) roasted tahini

1 teaspoon hazelnut butter

½ teaspoon local or raw honey or yacon syrup

3 tablespoons (45 ml) extra-virgin olive oil

1 tablespoon (9 g) capers, rinsed

3 tablespoons (45 ml) fresh lemon juice

Zest of 1 small organic lemon

8 teaspoons (40 ml) cold water

⅛ cup (28 ml) full-fat coconut milk

3 drops of Tabasco Red Pepper Sauce, or more if you prefer a hot sauce

1 pinch of each, or more to taste: sea salt, freshly ground pepper, ground ginger, cumin, and ground turmeric

1. In a small saucepan, sauté the shallot and garlic clove in a little bit of olive oil until translucent and fragrant.

2. Add all the ingredients to a blender, including the contents of the saucepan, and blend until creamy. If it needs more liquid, add a little bit more water or coconut milk.

3. Taste and season with more salt and pepper, lemon juice, and Tabasco Red Pepper Sauce if necessary.

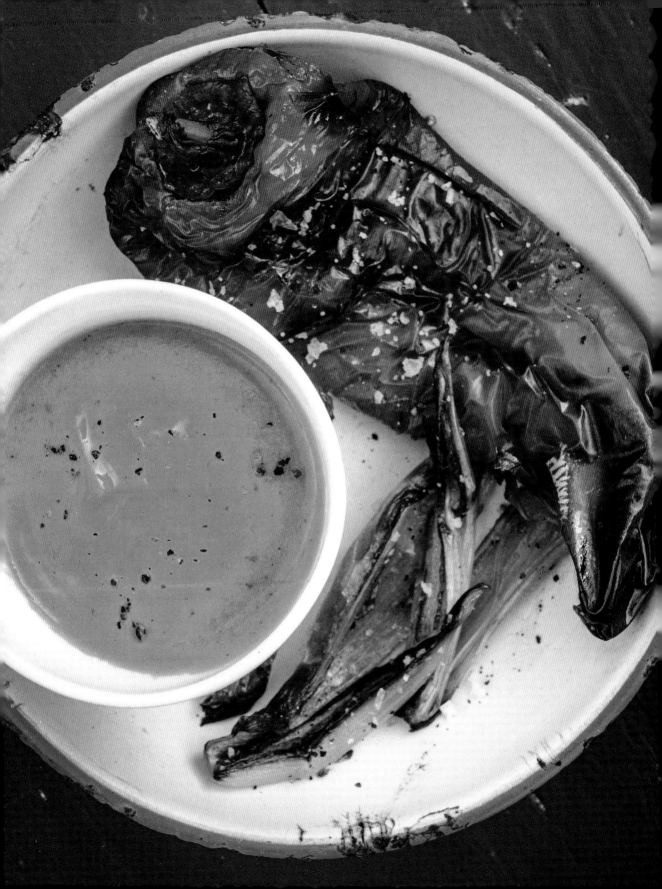

ROASTED RED PEPPER VINAIGRETTE

You can use it for eggs, chicken salad, sweet potato wedges, burgers, meatballs, or as a sauce for Buddha Bowls. This recipe includes roasting the peppers, peeling, and deseeding them, but you can also use the jarred ones. Just make sure you read the ingredients before buying.

Preparation time:
15 minutes

Cooking time:
30 minutes

Makes:
About ½ cup (120 ml)

2–3 red bell peppers

2 medium shallots, quartered or halved

3–4 garlic cloves, whole and unpeeled

1 tablespoon (15 ml) apple cider vinegar

5 tablespoons (75 ml) extra-virgin olive oil

4–5 tablespoons (60 to 75 ml) water, or more for thinner consistency

Pinch of salt

Pinch of freshly ground pepper

Optional: Tabasco Red Pepper Sauce

1. Preheat the oven to 400°F (200°C, or gas mark 6) and prepare a baking tray.

2. Add the bell peppers, shallots, and garlic to the baking tray. Bake until the peppers get soft and the skin blisters and the shallots get soft and develop brown spots, but not burnt. It can take up to 30 minutes, but you can take them out before if they are ready. Alternatively, you can roast the vegetables on a grill or a griddle.

3. Place the peppers into a bowl, generously sprinkle with salt, and cover. Let them rest for about 10 to 15 minutes. They'll soften up and the skin will be much easier to peel.

4. Peel and deseed the pepper and roughly chop them. Peel the garlic cloves.

5. Add all the ingredients, including the roasted shallots, to a high-powered blender and mix until creamy and smooth. If you want a thinner consistency or your blender requires more liquid, add a little more water.

6. Taste and add more apple cider vinegar, salt, and pepper if necessary.

7. If you want a kick, you can add a few drops of Tabasco Red Pepper Sauce.

BASIL AND ASPARAGUS PESTO WITH PISTACHIOS

Asparagus is one of my favorite vegetables. I love it for its nutritional value and taste, but also because it has antihistamine properties. Did you know that asparagus is a great source of prebiotics, plant protein, and even melatonin? The idea to use asparagus in a pesto came one day when I wanted to make a green sauce pizza and didn't have many greens in the refrigerator. I decided to try asparagus, and it was perfect. I love to use it for any pizza, especially the Asparagus Pies with Pomegranates on page 160.

Preparation time:
15 minutes

Makes:
About 1 cup
(260 g)

1 generous handful of basil leaves

About 10 asparagus spears (medium size), woody ends removed

¼ cup (60 ml) extra-virgin olive oil

¼ cup (31 g) raw pistachios

1 garlic clove

½ teaspoon salt

⅛ teaspoon freshly ground pepper

1–2 tablespoons (15 to 28 ml) fresh lemon juice to taste

Combine all the ingredients in a high-powered blender until creamy and smooth. Taste and adjust for salt and lemon juice if necessary. Use immediately or store in a jar in the fridge for a couple of days.

LECTIN-LIGHT KETCHUP

This recipe is inspired by the ketchup my mom makes every fall. She preserves it for the winter, but I rarely use ketchup, so I only make a small batch every now and then and store it for about 5 days in the refrigerator. The tomatoes are peeled and deseeded, and the peppers are previously roasted, which gives them a nice, smoky flavor and makes them very easy to peel. You can roast the peppers at home (page 74), or you can buy them jarred.

Preparation time:
15 minutes

Cooking time:
40 minutes

Makes:
About 1½ cups (260 g)

2 cups (360 g) peeled and deseeded tomatoes (fresh or from a can), blended

½ cup (90 g) roasted red peppers, peeled and deseeded, blended

1 teaspoon minced garlic

1 teaspoon prepared mustard

¼ teaspoon freshly ground pepper

2 bay leaves

Pinch of cinnamon

Pinch of nutmeg

½ to 1 teaspoon salt to taste

1 or 2 teaspoons inulin powder (or another sweetener), or to your taste

1 teaspoon apple cider vinegar

2 tablespoons (28 ml) extra-virgin olive oil

1 big onion, diced

1. Add the tomatoes to a medium saucepan and start cooking on low-to-medium heat until some of the water evaporates and they start to thicken.

2. Add the blended roasted red peppers, garlic, mustard, spices, sweetener, and apple cider vinegar. Continue to simmer on low heat.

3. Heat a skillet with olive oil and sauté the onions until they become golden brown.

4. Add the onions with the oil to the saucepan mixture and continue to simmer for about 10 more minutes or until it reaches your desired thickness.

5. Taste and adjust the spices and sweetener if necessary. Remove the bay leaves.

6. If you want a smooth consistency, you can blend everything in a blender.

7. Store in a jar in the fridge for up to 5 days. It can also be frozen in ice cube trays if you intend to use it in stews or pasta sauces.

DAIRY-FREE RANCH DRESSING

Making a white, creamy dressing or sauce when you don't eat dairy or cashews is not an easy feat. That's why I feel this dairy-free ranch dressing recipe is quite an accomplishment. It's really tasty, and it passed all the taste tests in our home. In this recipe, I used soaked blanched almonds, but an even easier way to make this dressing is to use blanched almond butter.

Preparation time:
15 minutes

Makes:
2 cups
(475 ml)

½ cup (73 g) blanched almonds (soaked)

½ cup (75 g) hemp seeds

1 garlic clove

2 tablespoons (20 g) chopped onion or 1 small shallot

1 small handful of fresh parsley

½ teaspoon dried chives

1 teaspoon dried dill

1 teaspoon salt

¼ teaspoon freshly ground pepper

½ cup (120 ml) filtered water

4–5 tablespoons (60 to 75 ml) extra-virgin olive oil

Juice of 1 lemon

1 tablespoon (15 ml) apple cider vinegar

1. To prepare the almonds: If your almonds are already blanched, soak them in cold water for about 5 hours. If your almonds are not blanched, to do so, soak the almonds with skins in water in the fridge for about 24 hours. After soaking, the skins will come off easily.

2. To make the dressing: Add the soaked almonds and all of the remaining ingredients to a blender and combine until creamy and smooth. You can add more water if it needs more liquid. Adjust the taste to your preference, adding more lemon juice, apple cider vinegar, salt, or pepper.

3. Store in a closed jar for up to 2 days in the fridge.

GREEN MANGO SALSA

An alternative to tomato salsa, green mango salsa is the perfect accompaniment for your tacos, but it really is more versatile than that. It adds a bright, fresh, sweet, and tangy touch to enchiladas, tostadas, nachos, and even steak or chicken.

Preparation time:
15 minutes

Makes:
1½ cups
(375 g)

1 green mango, peeled and cut into small cubes

1 scallion, finely chopped

1 handful of cilantro, washed, dried, and chopped

2 tablespoons (28 ml) extra-virgin olive oil

Juice of ½ lime, or more to taste

1 teaspoon apple cider vinegar, or more to taste

Pinch of salt to taste

Pinch of freshly ground pepper

A few drops of Tabasco Red Pepper Sauce to taste

Optional: a pinch of quality paprika, if you are not super sensitive to nightshades

Mix all the ingredients together, adjust the taste to your preference, and serve. Let the salsa sit in the fridge for a few hours before eating. The flavors will intensify, and it will become juicier.

POMEGRANATE REDUCTION

I started using pomegranate to make sauces and dressings when I had to start a low-histamine diet. Not only are pomegranates delicious and nutritious, but they also have antihistamine properties. I love using this reduction as an addition to meat sauces, to replace balsamic vinegar in salads, or to drizzle on meat and vegetables.

Preparation time:
15 minutes

Cooking time:
15 minutes

Makes:
About 1 cup
(235 ml)

Arils from 2 medium pomegranates

1 teaspoon inulin powder (or another sweetener)

1 whole clove

1. Blend the pomegranate arils in a high-powered blender and strain through a sieve, cheesecloth, or nut milk bag, making sure you get all the juices out.

2. Add the pomegranate juice, sweetener, and whole clove to a saucepan and simmer on low heat until it's reduced to half the quantity.

3. Store in a glass jar in the fridge for up to 3 days. Remove the clove before serving.

GREEN GARLIC SAUCE

If you like garlic on everything, try this sauce. It was inspired by a traditional Romanian garlic concoction, called *mujdei*, which is a mix of garlic, salt, and water and sometimes yogurt is added. It's perfect for fish and roasted vegetables, but it goes with anything.

Preparation time:
5 minutes

Makes:
About ½ cup (114 g)

3 spring garlic (green garlic) (if they are big, use less), chopped

4 tablespoons (60 ml) extra-virgin olive oil

¼ cup (60 ml) hemp milk, homemade (page 33) or store-bought (you can use any other compliant milk except for coconut milk)

1 teaspoon apple cider vinegar, or more to taste

Salt and freshly ground pepper to taste

1. Add the chopped garlic, olive oil, hemp milk, and apple cider vinegar to a blender.

2. Blend until smooth and add salt and pepper to taste.

BITTER GREENS PESTO WITH ARUGULA AND MÂCHE

"The bitter, the better," that's what **Dr. Steven Gundry says** when it comes to greens. While this pesto is a little stronger in taste, it is very healthy for us and an easy way to eat as much bitter greens as possible. I like to add it to eggs, or roasted vegetables, serve it with chicken or meat, or even use it as a pasta or pizza sauce.

Preparation time:
15 minutes

Makes:
About 1½ cups (336 g)

5 cups (100 g) arugula

2 cups (100 g) mâche (lamb's lettuce)

1 handful of basil leaves

2 garlic cloves, minced

3 tablespoons (30 g) pine nuts, toasted

Zest of 1 organic lemon

½ cup (120 ml) extra-virgin olive oil

2 tablespoons (28 ml) fresh lemon juice

¼–½ teaspoon salt (start with a smaller quantity and add to taste)

¼ teaspoon freshly ground pepper

Optional: ¼ cup (25 g) grated Parmigiano Reggiano

1. Process all the greens, garlic, pine nuts, and lemon zest in a food processor until minced. If necessary, stop and scrape the walls with a spatula.

2. With the food processor on low speed, start adding the olive oil.

3. Add the lemon juice, salt, and pepper and pulse until all the ingredients are combined.

4. Taste and adjust the salt, pepper, and lemon juice to your preference.

5. If you eat dairy, you can add Parmigiano Reggiano.

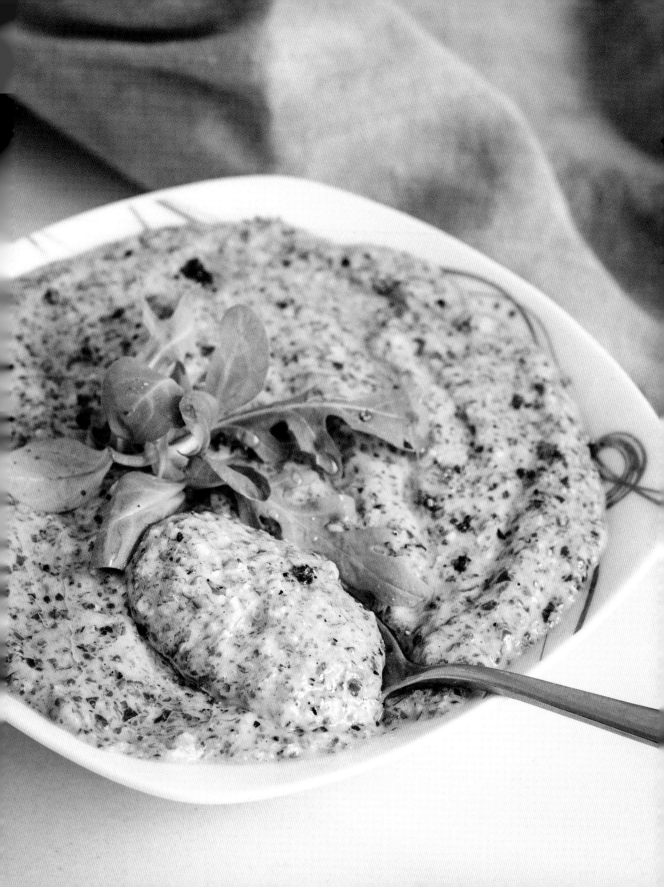

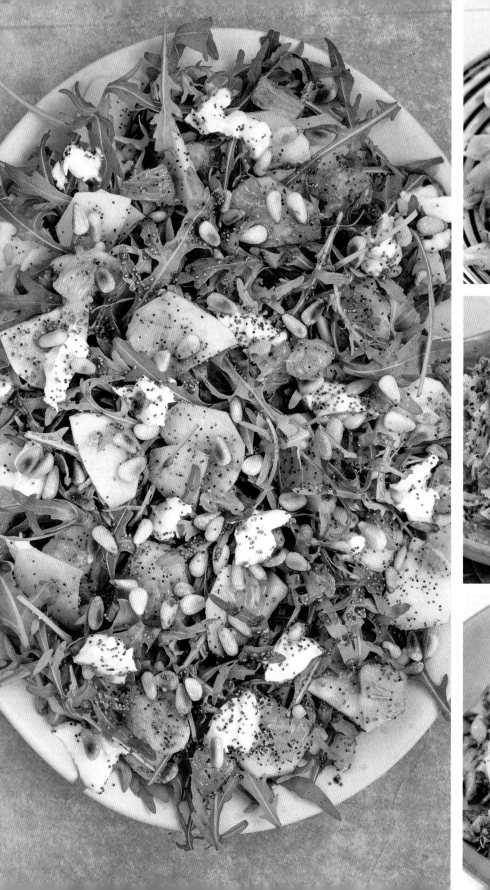
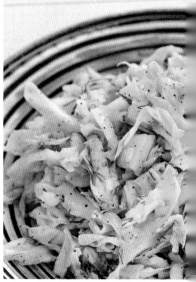
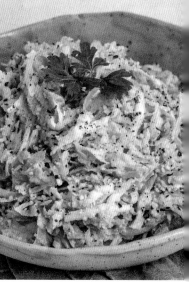
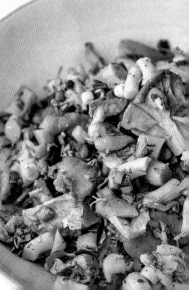

6

Salads

Clockwise from top left: Kohlrabi and Arugula Salad with Citrus and Buffalo Mozzarella (page 97); Cabbage Salad with Dill (page 102); Celeriac Slaw with Homemade Mayonnaise (page 101); Quick-Pickled Oyster Mushroom Salad (page 100)

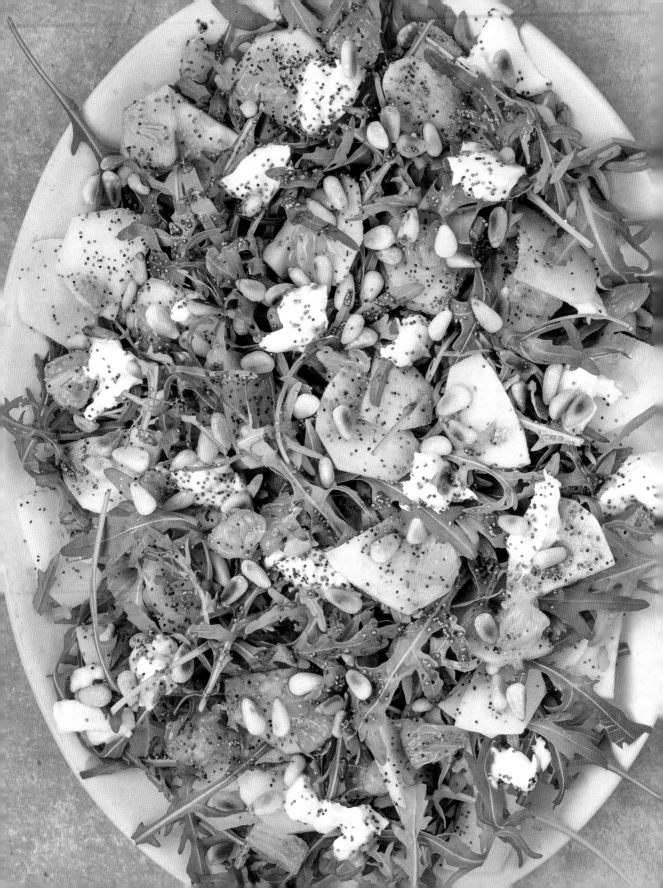

KOHLRABI AND ARUGULA SALAD WITH CITRUS AND BUFFALO MOZZARELLA

This salad is so easy to make and so delicious that it can be a regular item in your meal plans, but it's also quite sophisticated and makes a great salad on a holiday menu or to impress guests. It can be eaten as an appetizer or a side dish.

Preparation time:
20 minutes

Serves:
4

FOR THE BALSAMIC HONEY VINAIGRETTE:

1 tablespoon (15 ml) aged balsamic vinegar

3 tablespoons (45 ml) extra-virgin olive oil

⅛ teaspoon local or raw honey

Pinch of salt and freshly ground pepper

FOR THE SALAD:

2 tablespoons (20 g) pine nuts (a handful), toasted

4 cups (80 g) arugula (about 4 generous handfuls)

2 small kohlrabies, peeled

1 small clementine, or ½ orange

1 ball of buffalo mozzarella, shredded in small pieces

1 teaspoon poppy seeds

1. To make the balsamic honey vinaigrette: Whisk together all the ingredients. Set aside.

2. Toast the pine nuts in a pan on low heat for a few minutes until golden light brown blisters are formed. Transfer to a bowl and let them cool.

3. Arrange the arugula (washed and well dried) on a salad platter.

4. Halve the kohlrabi and then finely slice each half. Arrange on top of the arugula.

5. Peel the white skin from the clementine wedges and roughly chop them. Arrange on the platter.

6. Top with the shredded mozzarella pieces, toasted pine nuts, and poppy seeds.

7. Drizzle with balsamic honey vinaigrette to your taste and serve.

CHICKEN SALAD WITH HOMEMADE MAYONNAISE, POMEGRANATE, AND BASIL

This is a great way to use leftover chicken, or when you make a chicken broth using a whole chicken (page 106). In some parts of the world, it is difficult to find mayonnaise made with pastured eggs and a healthy oil, so I encourage you to make mayonnaise at home. It's actually very easy. Although it can be made quickly and effortlessly with an immersion blender if you use whole eggs, I only use egg yolks, and those need to be mixed by hand (an electric mixer might work too). Egg whites, if not cooked properly, can be high in histamine, and I prefer to keep my diet on the low histamine side. The recipe requires extra-virgin olive oil because I prefer it to avocado oil, but if you want a milder-tasting oil, you can certainly use avocado oil.

Preparation time:
30 minutes

Makes:
About 5 cups
(1 kg)

FOR THE MAYONNAISE:

2 pastured egg yolks

1 teaspoon Dijon mustard

About ½ cup (120 ml) extra-virgin olive oil (or avocado oil for a milder, more neutral taste)

1–2 tablespoons (15 to 28 ml) fresh lemon juice

Salt and freshly ground pepper to taste

FOR THE CHICKEN SALAD:

About 4 cups (900 g) shredded, cooked chicken

2 big celery ribs, finely sliced

Arils from 1 medium pomegranate

Salt and freshly ground pepper to taste

1 handful of fresh basil

1. To make the mayonnaise: Separate the egg yolks and add them to a mixing bowl with the mustard. Start combining with a wooden spoon, clockwise (don't change the direction), in a regular and consistent motion. With the other hand, slowly drizzle olive oil over the eggs and continue to mix in a circular motion. The consistency should become like a custard as you add more oil. When you finish the oil, add some lemon juice and continue to mix. Add salt and pepper, taste, and adjust to your preference.

2. Mix the mayonnaise with the rest of the ingredients. Add more salt and pepper if necessary. You can also add more Dijon mustard if you feel like it.

3. Serve with cassava tortillas, compliant toast, lettuce boats, or a green salad.

FATTOUSH SALAD, THE LECTIN-LIGHT WAY

Fattoush salad is traditionally made of many lectin-heavy vegetables and pita croutons. Fortunately, there are ways to prepare these vegetables to remove lectins and the pita croutons can be made using lectin-free tortillas. This fattoush salad is great as a tapas side dish, next to hummus, olives, and maybe some turkey or chicken meatballs (page 126).

Preparation time:
35 minutes

Serves:
2–4

FOR THE SALAD:

2 small cucumbers, peeled and seeds removed, sliced

1 medium heirloom tomato, peeled and seeds removed, cubed

1 small red onion, finely sliced

1 generous handful of purslane leaves or romaine heart (or both)

4–5 red radishes, sliced

1 small handful of chopped parsley

About 20 mint leaves, chopped, plus more for garnish

Fresh lemon juice to taste

Salt to taste

FOR THE DRESSING:

2 tablespoons (28 ml) extra-virgin olive oil

2 tablespoons (18 g) hemp seeds

2 tablespoons (28 ml) water, or more if necessary

1 garlic clove

1 teaspoon sumac

Juice of ½ lemon (or to your taste)

½ teaspoon salt

Freshly ground pepper

FOR THE PITA CROUTONS:

2 Easy Cassava Flour Tortillas (page 58) or any lectin-free tortillas

Extra-virgin olive oil

1. Prepare all the salad ingredients. Season the cucumbers and tomatoes with salt.

2. Make the croutons using cassava tortillas or any gluten-free and lectin-free tortillas you have, using one of the methods described in the sidebar below.

3. Make the dressing by blending all the ingredients in a blender until smooth and creamy.

4. Mix all the salad ingredients in a salad bowl and add a couple of tablespoons (28 to 45 ml) of dressing to the salad. Add half of the croutons to the salad bowl, combine, and taste. Add more dressing if necessary and season with salt and pepper to taste.

5. Add the rest of the croutons on top of the salad, drizzle with a little more dressing, and sprinkle with a little sumac powder and serve.

HOW TO MAKE PITA CROUTONS

This is easy. Traditionally, the croutons for fattoush salad are made with stale pitas that are fried in olive oil. Take a few cassava tortillas (page 58) or any other lectin-free tortillas, smother them with olive oil, and bake them in the oven or cook them in a cast-iron pan until crispy. Alternatively, you can first cut the soft tortillas into small squares, toss them with extra-virgin olive oil, and bake them until crispy, or you can even crisp them on a cast-iron pan or griddle. Choose the method that's easiest for you.

QUICK-PICKLED OYSTER MUSHROOM SALAD

I've always loved the texture and taste of pickled mushrooms. Combined with fresh herbs and spices, they make a nutritious and refreshing spring or summer salad or side dish. And quick-pickling the mushrooms is incredibly easy. One of the main reasons I decided to include this salad in the book is that my mom, who never eats mushrooms (it's a texture thing), not only ate it, but said she loved it.

Preparation time:
20 minutes

Cooking time:
30 minutes

Serves:
4–6

FOR THE PICKLED MUSHROOMS:

1 pound 2 ounces (500 g) oyster mushrooms, cleaned

2 quarts (2 L) water

¼ cup (60 ml) apple cider vinegar

3 bay leaves

1 teaspoon peppercorns

1 teaspoon mustard seeds

1 teaspoon coriander seeds

1 teaspoon salt

6 allspice berries

FOR THE SALAD:

1 handful of fresh parsley, chopped

3 spring onions

1 spring garlic (green garlic)

½ teaspoon salt (start with ¼ teaspoon and increase to your taste)

⅛ teaspoon freshly ground pepper

1 tablespoon (15 ml) apple cider vinegar

4 tablespoons (45 ml) extra-virgin olive oil

Fresh lemon juice to taste

1. Pickle the mushrooms a few hours before the meal is planned (or even 1 or 2 days in advance). Add the water to a big pot and add all the rest of the ingredients for pickling, except for the mushrooms. Bring to a boil.

2. While the water is heating, prepare the mushrooms. Separate the stems, cut off the hard ends, and wash well. Depending on how big your mushrooms are, try to slice them lengthwise, in strips, but not too small. When the water starts boiling, add the mushrooms, set the heat on low, and simmer for about 25 to 30 minutes.

3. Prepare a jar or a glass container with a lid. You will need to let the mushrooms cool before you use them for the salad. Plus, the extra time will allow them to marinate more.

4. After the mushrooms have simmered, turn the heat off and let them cool down a little. Place them into the jar or glass container, pour some of the liquid and spices over the top, and let cool. Once cold, store in the fridge for a few hours.

5. About 15 minutes before your meal, prepare all the ingredients for the salad. Wash the parsley, onions, and garlic and let them dry.

6. Take the mushrooms out, trying your best to separate them from the whole spices. Chop the mushrooms and the greens and mix them in a bowl.

7. Add all the rest of the ingredients, but add the salt gradually and taste. Squeeze more lemon juice if you want, and an extra drizzle of olive oil is always welcome.

8. Serve as a side salad, sandwich or taco filling, or include into a tapas-style meal.

CELERIAC SLAW WITH HOMEMADE MAYO

This has been one of my favorite salads since I was a child. You can serve it as a side dish with absolutely anything or use it for burger and sandwiches fillings. You can add some shredded chicken or salmon to it and make it your main dish. While you can use any compliant mayo you have, I love my homemade mayo, which is ready in just 8 minutes. Let this salad rest in the refrigerator for a few hours before serving.

Preparation time:
20 minutes

Serves:
2

2 cups (312 g) grated celeriac (celery root)

1 cup (110 g) grated carrots

1 very small green apple, grated

¼ cup (60 g) Basic Mayonnaise (page 29)

1 tablespoon (9 g) hemp seeds

Salt and freshly ground pepper to taste

Fresh lemon juice to taste

Fresh parsley for garnish

Mix everything together and serve or store in an airtight container for a few hours before serving.

CABBAGE SALAD WITH DILL

"No meals without a cabbage salad": that should be my family's motto. We've been eating this salad since we were kids, and no matter how big the salad is, we never have leftovers. It's my favorite low-carb side dish for stews, casseroles, all kind of meats, and even eggs. The secret to this salad's specific taste and texture is a fine shred and a good massage, as well as a cabbage head that is airy and light, not a dense and heavy one. While I love all kinds of cabbage, I would only use white cabbage (round or sugarloaf) for this salad.

Preparation time:
15 minutes

Serves:
4

1 cabbage head, finely shredded

½–1 teaspoon salt

2–3 tablespoons (28 to 45 ml) extra-virgin olive oil

1–2 tablespoons (15 to 28 ml) apple cider vinegar

Freshly ground pepper

1 bunch fresh dill, finely chopped

1. Finely shred the cabbage on a work surface, sprinkle ½ teaspoon salt on it, and massage until the fibers start to break and juices start to come out.

2. Transfer to a big serving bowl, gradually add the olive oil and apple cider vinegar, pepper, and dill, and combine well.

3. Taste and season with more salt or vinegar if necessary. Usually different people have different preferences, especially when it comes to salt and vinegar. Some like it more sour, while others like it more sweet. You can always add some apple cider vinegar to your plate if necessary.

BITTER GREENS BISTRO SALAD

A bistro salad is the typical green salad you get next to a quiche in a French restaurant. I don't know about you, but I couldn't eat that quiche, or anything with eggs, without a salad. I'm known for doubling or tripling my green salad order. Sometimes, if you are lucky, you can find a bistro salad mix in stores, already washed, and you can certainly use that to make the salad, or you can make your own mix. The serving size is just a suggestion. I often eat it all just by myself.

Preparation time:
5 minutes

Serves:
2–4

1 generous handful of radicchio, shredded

1 generous handful of endives, roughly chopped

1 generous handful of romaine lettuce

1 generous handful of arugula

¼ cup (60 ml) Basic Balsamic Vinaigrette (page 30)

Layer all the salad leaves in a bowl and mix with the dressing. Serve immediately.

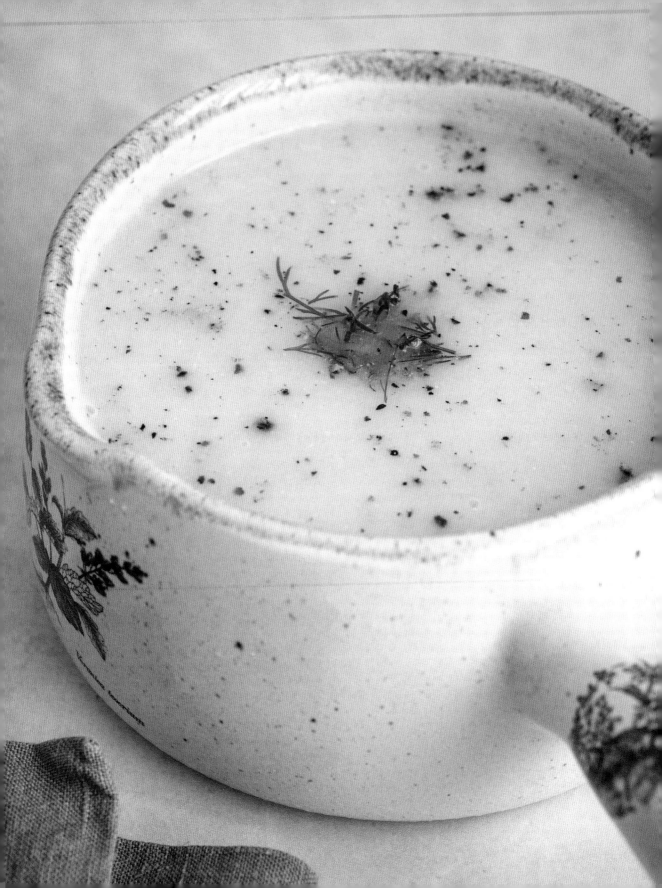

7

Soups

LEFTOVER-CHICKEN BROTH AND CHICKEN SOUP

After you make whole roasted chicken, use all the leftover bones and carcass, and even the liquid and the veggies, to make a delicious chicken broth or even a soup. This recipe is made in a pressure cooker and is super easy. If you make just a broth, store it in jars in the refrigerator or freeze it for later use. If you have chicken left and want to make a chicken soup, just add some fresh vegetables to the broth, some shredded chicken, and maybe some millet noodles and in 15 minutes, you have a chicken soup.

Preparation time:
30 minutes

Cooking time:
25 minutes

Serves:
4–6

FOR THE BROTH:

1 chicken carcass, left over from roasting a whole chicken, plus any bones, skins, juices, and vegetables left

1 yellow onion, cut in half

1 big carrot

1 parsnip

1 big piece celeriac (celery root)

2 celery ribs

½ fennel bulb

3 garlic cloves, whole

1 thumb-size piece of fresh gingerroot

1 thumb-size piece of fresh turmeric root

2 sprigs fresh thyme

1 teaspoon black peppercorns

2 bay leaves

1 teaspoon salt

1 tablespoon (15 ml) apple cider vinegar

1 small bunch parsley

Water (to cover the contents)

FOR THE SOUP:

1–2 carrots, sliced or cut any shape you want

1 parsnip, sliced or chopped

2 celery ribs, finely sliced

1 piece of celeriac (celery root), chopped

½ fennel bulb, chopped

1 big bunch fresh parsley, chopped

2–3 cups (450 to 675 g) shredded leftover chicken

Salt and freshly ground pepper to taste

Optional: millet noodles (or other lectin-free pasta)

1. Add the carcass, any leftovers you have from roasting the chicken, the fresh vegetables, and the rest of the ingredients to the pressure cooker. The vegetables should be in big chunks or whole. Pressure cook for 15 minutes and allow the pressure to release naturally. At this point, you can store the broth in the fridge for up to 3 days or freeze for future use, or you can continue and make a chicken soup.

2. Strain the broth and return back to the heat. Add all the chopped vegetables minus the parsley and boil for about 10 to 15 minutes until the vegetables are tender.

3. At the end, add the fresh parsley and the leftover chicken. Season with salt and pepper to taste and serve.

4. You can also add millet noodles (or other lectin-free pasta) along with the vegetables, if desired.

CREAMY VEGETABLE SOUP WITH BUTTERNUT SQUASH (or Sweet Potato)

Squashes are fruits, not vegetables, so the fruit rule applies here. Have some only occasionally and in season. My favorite way to have squash is as a creamy soup. I use a pressure cooker to speed the cooking time, but also to remove lectins. If not in season, you can replace the squash with sweet potato.

Preparation time:
30 minutes

Cooking time:
20 minutes

Serves:
4

3–4 tablespoons (45 to 60 ml) extra-virgin olive oil

1 yellow onion, chopped

2 leeks, the white part, chopped

1 parsnip, chopped

1 carrot, chopped

2 sticks celery, chopped

1 small celeriac (celery root), chopped (about ½ cup [78 g])

4–5 cauliflower florets

½ butternut squash, seeds removed and peeled, cubed (replace with sweet potato when squash is not in season)

2 cloves garlic, smashed and chopped

2 sprigs fresh thyme or ¼ teaspoon dried

2 teaspoons salt, or more to taste

⅛ teaspoon freshly ground pepper

⅛ teaspoon nutmeg

⅛ teaspoon ground mustard

1½ quarts (1.5 L) hot water

Optional: organic cream or coconut cream, fresh thyme leaves, freshly ground pepper, or croutons

1. Heat the olive oil in your pressure cooker on medium heat or use the sauté option if available.

2. Add all the chopped veggies, minus the squash. Stir occasionally and let them sauté for about 10 minutes until the vegetables soften and become fragrant, without browning them.

3. In the meantime, you can prepare the squash.

4. Add the spices and the squash, stir well, and cook for 1 to 2 more minutes.

5. Add the water, bring to a boil, and pressure cook for 5 minutes. Let the pressure release naturally.

6. Blend the soup in a blender or with a stick blender until creamy and bring it back to a boil.

7. You can serve it as is or add a little bit of cream or coconut cream. Garnish with fresh thyme, pepper, and croutons if you like.

MEATBALL SOUR SOUP, ROMANIAN STYLE

Meatball soup is a staple of many culinary traditions, and Romanian cuisine is not an exception. I grew up with this soup, and I love making it every now and then. Usually this requires a longer cooking time, but now we make it in a pressure cooker, which shortens the cooking time and also makes it possible to use rice, tomato, red pepper, and even potato. Traditionally, the meatballs are made with ground pork, but you can use chicken, turkey, or beef or a mix.

Preparation time:
35 minutes

Cooking time:
40 minutes

Serves:
8

FOR THE MEATBALLS:

1 pound (455 g) finely ground pork, 10% fat (can be replaced with chicken, turkey, or beef or a mix)

1 pastured egg

1 small onion, grated

1 tablespoon (12 g) Indian basmati rice, rinsed well, uncooked

1 teaspoon salt

1 teaspoon freshly ground pepper

FOR THE SOUP:

1 tomato, peeled and deseeded, chopped

1 big carrot, chopped

1 big parsnip, chopped

1 leek, chopped

1 onion, grated

½ small celeriac (celery root), chopped

3 celery ribs, chopped

1 red bell pepper, seeds removed and peeled, with a vegetable peeler, chopped

2 white potatoes, peeled and cubed, bigger size than the rest of the veggies (can be skipped)

1 teaspoon salt

¼ teaspoon freshly ground pepper

Souring agent: Borscht, apple cider vinegar, fresh lemon juice, or sauerkraut juice, to your taste

FOR SERVING:

Fresh lovage or parsley

Optional: organic sour cream

---

1. Peel and deseed the tomato and chop all the vegetables.

2. Add about 3 quarts (3 L) of water to your pressure cooker, add the vegetables, and bring to a boil (don't add the lid yet).

3. In a bowl, mix well the minced pork with the egg, onion, rice, salt, and pepper. Shape into small balls (the size that can fit in the spoon you will serve the soup with), making sure there is no air left inside or cracks on the surface.

4. When the liquid is boiling, add the meatballs one by one to the boiling soup. Add more salt and pepper (you can always add more later).

5. Close the lid of the pressure cooker and pressure cook for about 40 minutes.

6. Release the pressure and adjust for spices and add the souring liquid you are using. Add gradually and taste.

7. Add fresh lovage or parsley to the pot and serve. If you eat dairy, you can serve the soup with a dollop of organic sour cream.

BLACK BEAN SOUP

Inspired by one of my favorite Romanian bean soups, this soup, served with smashed and salted red onion and a piece of Super Easy Focaccia Bread (page 54), is truly comfort food for me. If you prefer, you can make it thicker so it is more like a stew.

Preparation time:
20 minutes

Cooking time:
1 hour

Serves:
4–5

3–4 tablespoons (45 to 60 ml) extra-virgin olive oil

1 big yellow onion, chopped

½ fennel bulb, sliced

1 carrot, chopped

2 celery ribs, finely sliced

1 red bell pepper, peels and seeds removed, chopped or sliced

1 teaspoon salt, or more to taste

¼ teaspoon freshly ground pepper

1 bay leaf

3 cups (516 g) soaked and pressure cooked black beans (or use canned black beans, drained and rinsed)

Warm water to cover all the vegetables

1 handful of fresh parsley, chopped

FOR SERVING:

1 red onion, smashed and salted in advance

Super Easy Focaccia Bread (page 54)

1. Pour the olive oil in a thick pot or deep pan and when hot, add the onion, fennel, carrot, celery, and bell pepper. Sauté on low-to-medium heat for about 10 minutes, stirring occasionally, until the vegetables soften. Don't brown them. If necessary, lower the heat or add a little bit of water to the pan.

2. Add the salt, pepper, bay leaf, and beans and cover with warm water. Simmer on low-to-medium heat for about 45 minutes. Make sure there is always enough water, adding more if necessary. The consistency should be like a thin stew, but you can also adapt it to your taste, adding more water or less. Keep in mind that will also thicken further when cooled.

3. Remove the bay leaf before serving.

4. Finish with fresh parsley and more salt and pepper if necessary.

5. You can serve this soup immediately, or you can keep in the fridge for up to 2 days and reheat when needed, next to a smashed and salted red onion, if you like raw onion, and a few slices of focaccia.

CREAMY LEEK AND KOHLRABI SOUP WITH MISO PASTE

Here's an unexpected combination of ingredients that work magic to create this creamy, light, but flavorful soup. Also, it's one of my favorite ways to use kohlrabi. If you can't find kohlrabi, you can replace it with cauliflower. They are in fact both from the cruciferous family, so they have similar health benefits and nutritional profile.

Preparation time:
15 minutes

Cooking time:
25 minutes

Serves:
4

3 leeks, green part removed, washed well and sliced

4 medium kohlrabies, peeled and cubed

1 medium parsnip, cut into small pieces

3 tablespoons (45 ml) extra-virgin olive oil

1 teaspoon grated ginger

1 teaspoon salt

¼ teaspoon freshly ground pepper

¼ teaspoon ground mustard

1 quart (1 L) hot water

4 tablespoons (60 g) coconut cream

1 tablespoon (16 g) white miso paste

Juice of ½ lime, or more to taste

Fresh dill or cilantro to serve

1. Sauté the leeks, kohlrabi, and parsnip on medium heat in the olive oil until the vegetables become fragrant and the leeks soften (don't brown anything), about 8 minutes, stirring frequently. Add the ginger and continue to cook for about 2 minutes.

2. Add the salt, pepper, and ground mustard and pour in the hot water. Bring to a boil and let everything simmer for about 10 minutes or until the kohlrabi and parsnip become fork-tender.

3. Take off the heat and blend everything (in a blender or with an immersion blender) until creamy.

4. Put back on the heat, add the coconut cream, and simmer for about 5 minutes.

5. Turn the heat off and add the miso paste, stirring well. Add the lime juice, taste, and add more salt if necessary.

6. Serve with fresh dill or cilantro and a squeeze of lime.

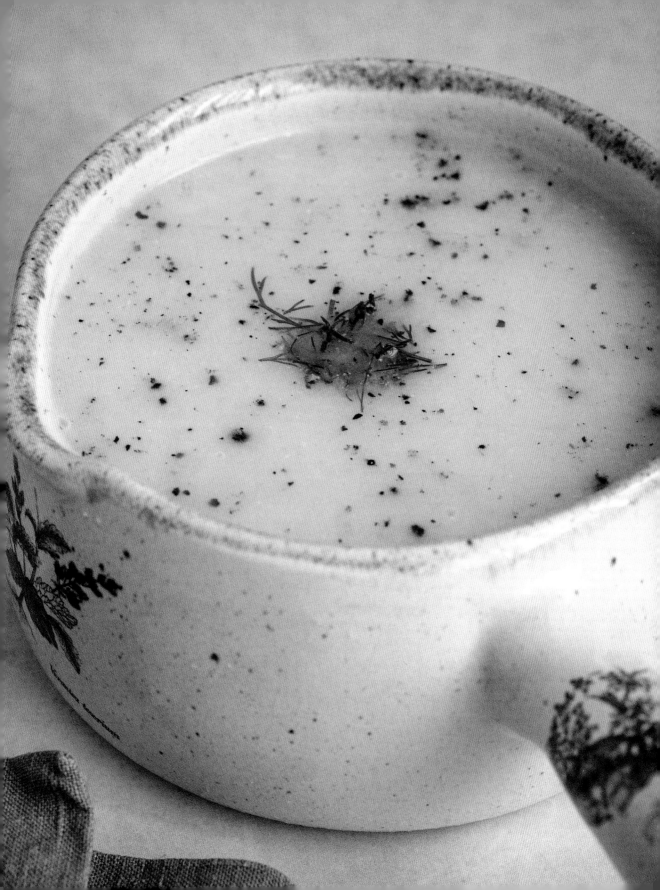

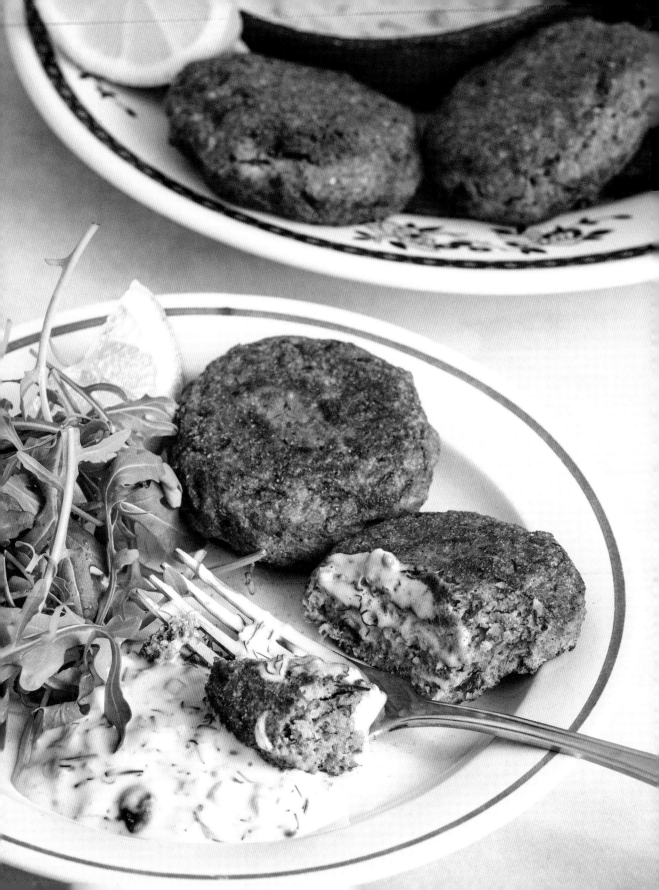

8

Main Courses with Fish and Seafood

Clockwise from top left: Danish-Style Fish Cakes with Dill-Yogurt Sauce (page 118)

GREEN CURRY SOUP WITH BAKED TURMERIC COD

This soup is easy to make, silky, and light but so delicious and satisfying. Look for a good-quality green curry paste. They are made through a fermentation process, hence acceptable for a lectin-light diet.

Preparation time:
20 minutes

Cooking time:
20 minutes

Serves:
2

FOR THE SOUP:

1 tablespoon (14 g) coconut oil

3 cups (213 g) chopped broccoli

3 cups (210 g) chopped bok choy

½ stick of lemongrass, smashed (see Note)

1 teaspoon green curry paste

1 can (13.5 ounces, or 380 g) full-fat coconut milk

⅞ cup (200 ml) water

½ teaspoon salt

⅛ teaspoon freshly ground pepper

1 handful of fresh cilantro

FOR THE FISH:

12½ ounces (350 g) fresh cod loin

½ teaspoon salt

¼ teaspoon freshly ground pepper

1 teaspoon ground turmeric

1 tablespoon (15 ml) extra-virgin olive oil

Juice of 1 lime

Salt and freshly ground pepper to taste

Optional: Tabasco Red Pepper Sauce

1. Preheat the oven to 350°F (180°C, or gas mark 4) and prepare a small baking tray for the fish. Prepare all the vegetables.

2. Rinse the fish and pat dry and place onto the baking tray. Season with salt, pepper, and turmeric, drizzle with olive oil, and bake for 15 to 20 minutes until white throughout and flaky. The time will depend on the thickness of the fish.

3. While the cod cooks, heat the coconut oil in a soup pot on medium heat.

4. Add the broccoli, bok choy, lemongrass stick, and curry paste and sauté for about 5 minutes until the veggies are vibrant green and the flavors come through.

5. Add the coconut milk and water, salt, and pepper and bring to a boil. Simmer on medium heat for 6 minutes. Remove the lemongrass stick, making sure there are not any woody parts left in the soup. (See Note.)

6. Transfer the contents to a blender, along with the fresh cilantro. If you have a glass blender, you can mix it warm. If you have a plastic one, wait until the soup cools down (so you might have to do this step before the fish). Blend until creamy and smooth.

7. Transfer the creamy soup back to the pot, reheat to serve, and season with lime juice and salt and pepper to taste.

8. To serve, split the soup into two bowls and add the flaky cod on top. Garnish with fresh cilantro, lime, and pepper. If you want more spice, you can add a few drops of Tabasco Red Pepper Sauce.

NOTE: To release all the flavors in the lemongrass, smash it before adding it to the pan. To make sure it doesn't break apart, leave one of the ends intact. You don't want the woody parts ending up in the soup.

CREAMY SHRIMP WITH LICORICE AND PARSLEY

This is my favorite way of eating shrimp. I love the subtle anise flavor and the creaminess and richness of the sauce. Pure licorice powder has amazing health benefits and is great for both sweet and savory dishes. Using small whole shrimp is the best for this dish, but if you don't like whole shrimp, keep the tail on and use a couple of whole shrimp during the cooking process for more flavor. This is an "eat with your hands and get messy" kind of dish, at least if you use whole shrimp.

Preparation time:
30 minutes

Cooking time:
15 minutes

Serves:
2

20 whole small shrimp, wild caught (head and shell on)

3–4 tablespoons (45 to 60 ml) extra-virgin olive oil

4 garlic cloves, minced

1 teaspoon grated ginger

1 teaspoon licorice powder or 1 shot (1.5 ounces [42 ml]) of sambuca liqueur

1 can (13.5 ounces, or 380 g) full-fat coconut milk

1 teaspoon salt

¼ teaspoon freshly ground pepper

1 teaspoon tapioca flour dissolved in 2 tablespoons (28 ml) cold water

1 heaping cup (60 g) chopped fresh parsley

Juice of 1 lemon

FOR SERVING:

Pressure cooked and cooled Indian basmati rice or cauliflower rice

A mixed green salad

1. Prepare the shrimp by rinsing them in cold water and patting them dry. If you want them deveined, ask your fish monger to do it without removing the shell and head. For the best flavor, keep the shell and head on, but if that's not your thing or you want the eating to be less messy, this can also work with peeled shrimp, even butterflied. They'll just have to cook less.

2. Heat the olive oil in a big skillet and arrange the shrimp so they don't overlap. Cook them on medium heat until pink, about 2 to 3 minutes. Flip them one by one on the other side and cook for 2 to 3 more minutes.

3. Add the garlic and ginger and cook and stir for about 3 minutes. If you are using the sambuca liqueur instead of licorice powder, now is the time to deglaze the pan with the shot of sambuca. Stir well.

4. Add the coconut milk, salt and pepper, and the licorice powder if using and bring to a simmer. Simmer on low heat for about 5 minutes.

5. For more thickness, add the tapioca flour and water mixture. Stir well and simmer for 1 more minute.

6. Turn off the heat and add the parsley and lemon juice to taste. Add more salt and pepper if necessary.

7. Serve with pressure cooked Indian basmati rice or cauliflower rice and/or a mixed green salad.

FISH AND CHIPS WITH PEA MASH

Fish fingers, fries, and pea mash are a staple in many pubs and one of my favorite dishes to order. Most of the time I would not eat the coating of the fish, as I found it too thick and greasy. I didn't like the taste of it, but I also knew it was soaked in seed oils. I have good news. There is a healthier way to cook and enjoy this staple, and it's not complicated at all. Pressure cooking the peas is essential to make this dish lectin-light.

Preparation time:
40 minutes

Cooking time:
40–45 minutes

Serves:
4

FOR THE CHIPS:

2 sweet potatoes

Salt and freshly ground pepper

FOR THE PEA MASH:

1 pound (455 g) frozen peas

2 shallots, finely chopped

1–2 tablespoons (15 to 28 ml) extra-virgin olive oil

1 teaspoon salt

¼ teaspoon freshly ground pepper

2 tablespoons (28 ml) extra-virgin olive oil

2 tablespoons (30 g) coconut cream

1 small handful of fresh mint leaves

Fresh lemon juice to taste

FOR THE FISH:

14 ounces (400 g) cod fish fillets

Salt and freshly ground pepper

2 tablespoons (18 g) sorghum flour

2 tablespoons (18 g) cassava flour

2 pastured eggs

Sea salt flakes for finishing

1–2 teaspoons malt vinegar

1. To make the pea mash: Add the frozen peas to a pressure cooker, cover with water, and pressure cook for 3 minutes. Allow the pressure to release for about 5 minutes and then release manually what's left.

2. In a skillet, sauté the shallots in the olive oil until soft. Add the drained peas, season with the salt and pepper, and sauté for 3 minutes. Transfer all to a blender and add the rest of the ingredients and blend until creamy. I like to retain a little bit of texture, so I don't overmix.

3. To make the chips: Preheat the oven to 400°F (200°C, or gas mark 6). Wash and scrub the potatoes, pat dry, and cut into wedges. Arrange them on a large baking sheet and put them in the oven (don't season yet).

4. To make the fish: While the potatoes are cooking, rinse and pat dry the cod fillets. Portion them into smaller size pieces. (I like them in the shape of fish fingers.) Generously season with salt and pepper.

5. Mix the flours on a plate and beat the eggs in a bowl. Dredge the fish in the flour mix, dip in the egg, and dredge again in the flour mix.

6. When they are all ready, make some space on the sheet pan with the potatoes, flip the potato wedges, and add the fish. Cook for about 15 more minutes. The potatoes and fish should be ready at about the same time (in total, the potato wedges need about 35 to 40 minutes).

7. Let everything rest for 5 minutes before serving. Generously season with sea salt flakes and pepper. Drizzle the malt vinegar on the fish fingers.

CREAMY SALMON WITH LEEKS, CAULIFLOWER, AND DAIKON RADISH

A very easy and quick weeknight dinner, this salmon dish with Chinese five-spice is healthy, comforting, and tasty. It's a mixture of a fish soup and a stew, and although I haven't tried, I'm sure it will work with other fish or seafood. Make sure the cauliflower is finely sliced so it doesn't take long to cook, or you can even use frozen cauliflower rice. This dish goes with anything pickled, and you can use the other half of the daikon radish to make some Quick Pickled Daikon Radish (page 31).

Preparation time:
15 minutes

Cooking time:
15–20 minutes

Serves:
4

2 leeks, white and green parts, chopped or sliced

2–3 tablespoons (28 to 45 ml) extra-virgin olive oil or avocado oil

2 garlic cloves, smashed and chopped

½ head medium cauliflower, florets finely sliced

½ daikon radish, cut into small cubes

1 teaspoon salt

¼ teaspoon freshly ground pepper

3 wild-caught salmon fillets (about 4½ ounces [125 g] each)

1 teaspoon Chinese five-spice mix

1 can (13.5 ounces, or 380 g) full-fat coconut milk

1 teaspoon tapioca flour dissolved in 2 tablespoons (28 ml) cold water

Juice of 1 lime

1. Sauté the leeks in olive oil in a large skillet until soft, about 8 minutes, stirring occasionally.

2. Add the garlic, cauliflower, daikon, salt, and pepper, mix well, and sauté for about 5 more minutes.

3. Make space in the pan and add the three salmon fillets, sprinkle them with half of the five-spice, cover, and cook for 2 to 3 minutes.

4. Flip the salmon, add the rest of the five-spice, and cook for 2 more minutes.

5. Break the salmon into flakes, add the coconut milk, and bring to a boil.

6. Add the tapioca and water mixture, simmer for 2 more minutes, and turn the heat off.

7. Add lime juice to taste and salt and pepper to finish.

8. This pairs beautifully with Quick Pickled Daikon Radish (page 31).

DANISH-STYLE FISH CAKES WITH DILL-YOGURT SAUCE

These fish cakes are inspired by the famous Danish *fiskefrikadeller*, a fish cake with a very fine texture, usually made with cod and served with Danish remoulade. I made a similar sauce, but simpler. Sometimes, I use a mix of cod and wild salmon, but only cod would work too. For this recipe I experimented with acorn flour, mixed with cassava, but any flour mix would work. You can keep it very low carb by using a nut flour, all except coconut flour.

Preparation time:
40 minutes

Cooking time:
20 minutes

Makes:
10 fish cakes

FOR THE SAUCE:

7 tablespoons (98 g) Basic Mayonnaise (page 29)

7 tablespoons (105 g) unsweetened goat, buffalo, or coconut yogurt

2 tablespoons (18 g) capers, rinsed, dried, and chopped

2 tablespoons (8 g) chopped dill

1 teaspoon grated onion

A squeeze of lemon

Pinch of salt if necessary (taste before, as some other elements are already salty)

Pinch of freshly ground pepper

FOR THE FISH CAKES:

14 ounces (400 g) total white fish fillet, like cod, and salmon fillet (you can use a 1:1 ratio)

1 medium onion, grated

1 pastured egg

2 tablespoons (30 g) coconut cream

Zest of 1 organic lemon

½ teaspoon salt

⅛ teaspoon freshly ground pepper

½ teaspoon curry powder

½ teaspoon ground allspice

2 tablespoons (8 g) chopped dill

5–8 tablespoons (weight will vary) flour (any lectin-free mix you have will work: cassava, hazelnut, almond, tigernut, etc.)

A generous amount of extra-virgin olive oil or avocado oil

FOR SERVING:

Big green salad

---

1. To make the sauce: Mix all the ingredients and keep refrigerated until the fish cakes are ready.

2. Cut the fish into cubes and mince in a food processor. We are looking for a paste-like texture, so don't be afraid to process well.

3. Add the onion, egg, coconut cream, lemon zest, and spices and process again until it is all incorporated.

4. Add about 4 tablespoons of lectin-free flour (weight will vary), pulse a few times, and transfer the paste to a mixing bowl.

5. Now, start adding more flour until you get a consistency that keeps the paste-like texture but is not too wet. The quantity and the color of the texture will depend on what flour you will use. When I took these pictures, the flour I used was cassava with acorn flour (which is dark brown), hence the dark color of the patties.

6. Make 10 patties.

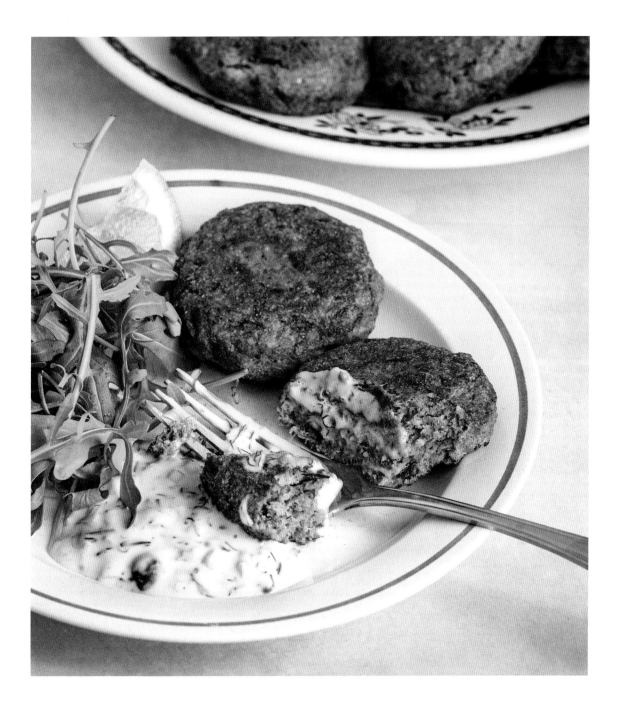

7. Add a generous amount of olive or avocado oil to a large skillet (about ⅛ inch [3 mm] deep) on medium heat. When hot, add as many patties as you can fit, without crowding the pan. I usually need to make them in two batches.

8. Fry for about 4 to 5 minutes per side, adjusting the heat if necessary. I like to keep it medium to low.

9. Serve the fish cakes with the sauce and a big green salad on the side.

SCALLOP TACOS WITH GREEN MANGO SALSA AND BUFFALO BURRATA

Who doesn't love tacos? While I do appreciate all types of tacos, sometimes I want something a little more special. Scallops are easy and fast to cook, and the rest of the elements of this dish take just a little bit of planning. Make a big batch of cassava tortillas when you have time and freeze them. Or, an even faster alternative, use store-bought lectin-free tortillas (no, that's not cheating!). Make the Green Mango Salsa (page 89) during the day when you have 10 minutes available and store it in the refrigerator until mealtime.

Preparation time:
40 minutes

Cooking time:
5 minutes

Serves:
4

FOR THE SCALLOPS:

1 pound (455 g) wild-caught scallops

¼ teaspoon salt

⅛ teaspoon freshly ground pepper

½ teaspoon cumin

½ teaspoon paprika

½ teaspoon ground allspice

1 tablespoon (15 ml) extra-virgin olive oil

1 tablespoon (14 g) grass-fed butter

2 garlic cloves, smashed

Juice of ½ lime

FOR ASSEMBLING THE TACOS:

8 Easy Cassava Flour Tortillas (page 58)

Cooked scallops, roughly chopped or sliced

1½ cups (375 g) Green Mango Salsa (made from 1 mango, page 89)

1 cup (70 g) shredded red cabbage

1 red onion, finely sliced

6 red radishes, finely sliced

1 buffalo burrata (or mozzarella if you can't find burrata), shredded

1 handful of fresh cilantro leaves

1 lime, cut into wedges

Optional: avocado, finely chopped or sliced

---

1. Before you cook the scallops, prepare all the filling ingredients and arrange them on a serving platter or individual plates. The mango salsa could be made in advance and kept in the fridge until the scallops are ready. The burrata should be shredded in small pieces.

2. Tortillas can be kept in the warm oven for a few minutes before the scallops are ready.

3. Clean and pat dry the scallops.

4. Mix all the spices, including the salt, in a bowl. Sprinkle the scallops on both sides with the spice mix.

5. Heat a cast-iron pan (or nonstick) on medium-to-high heat. Add the olive oil and butter and the smashed garlic cloves. When hot, add the scallops.

6. Sear for about 3 minutes on one side, without touching them, until golden brown. Flip and cook for 1 to 2 more minutes. They should be springy, not firm.

7. Remove them from the pan and place on a cutting board.

8. Drizzle them with lime juice and let rest for a minute. Then, chop or slice and add to the serving platter or individual plates.

9. Start with shredded red cabbage and continue with the rest of the ingredients in the order you prefer.

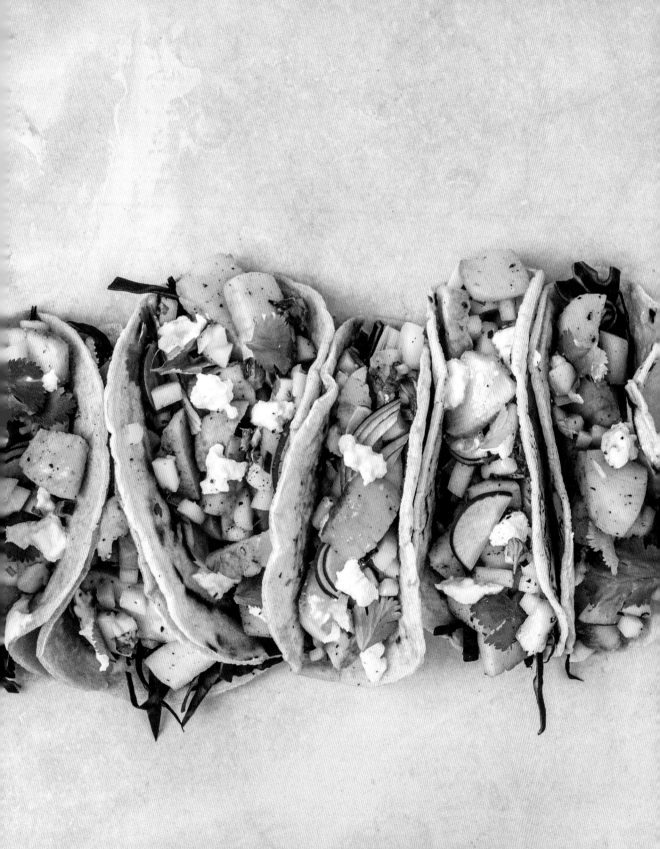

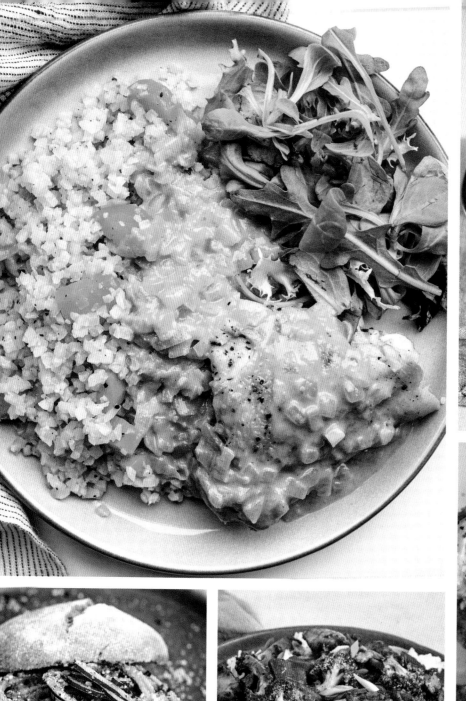
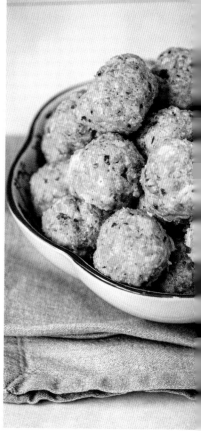
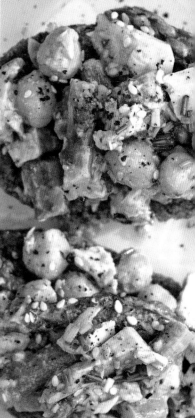
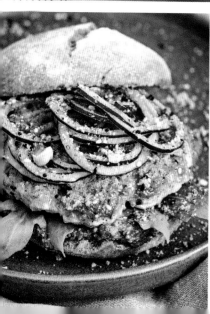
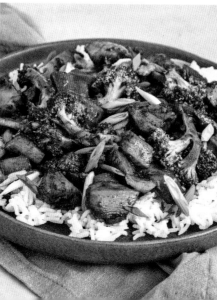

9

Main Courses with Chicken or Turkey

Clockwise from top left: Yellow Chicken Curry with Cauliflower Rice (page 136); Turkey Meatballs with Sorghum Spaghetti and Pesto (page 126); Chicken-Tahini Salad with Chickpeas and Asparagus (page 129); Kung Pao-Style Chicken and Broccoli (page 124); Turkey Burger with Dukkah Spice Mix and Pesto (page 130)

KUNG PAO–STYLE CHICKEN AND BROCCOLI

While this meal is inspired by the famous Kung Pao Chicken, it's not exactly the same thing, as it is adapted to fit a lectin-light lifestyle. Peanuts are replaced with macadamia nuts, there is no soy sauce or sugar, and this dish is not spicy (but you can add Tabasco Red Pepper Sauce). I added broccoli to make it more nutritionally balanced, but I kept the bell pepper, which I peel and deseed, as I think it is essential for the taste. Even if it is not as intense as the original recipe, it's a quick and easy comfort meal. I serve it with pressure cooked and cooled Indian basmati rice.

Preparation time:
30 minutes

Cooking time:
20 minutes

Serves:
2

FOR THE CHICKEN MARINADE:

2 servings of chicken breasts (about 10 ounces [280 g])

⅓ cup (80 ml) water

1 tablespoon (15 ml) rice vinegar

1 tablespoon (8 g) tapioca flour

1 tablespoon (15 ml) coconut aminos

1 tablespoon (15 ml) yacon syrup

2 teaspoons Dijon mustard

FOR THE DISH:

1 red bell pepper, peeled and deseeded

2 generous handfuls of broccoli florets, finely sliced

4 big garlic cloves, smashed and finely chopped

1 generous (8 g) tablespoon grated ginger

½ cup (68 g) raw macadamia nuts, roughly chopped

2–4 scallions (depending on how big they are), sliced

1 tablespoon (15 ml) coconut aminos

1 tablespoon (15 ml) rice vinegar

¼ cup (60 ml) water

1 tablespoon (15 ml) yacon syrup

2–3 (28 to 45 ml) tablespoons extra-virgin olive oil, avocado oil, or sesame oil

Salt and freshly ground pepper if necessary

FOR SERVING:

2 cups (316 g) pressure cooked and cooled Indian basmati rice (prepare one day in advance, cool overnight, and reheat)

Optional: Tabasco Red Pepper Sauce

---

1. Prepare the chicken and make the marinade. Cut the chicken breasts into bite-size pieces. Combine all the marinade ingredients and pour over the chicken. Cover and store in the fridge while you prepare the rest of the ingredients.

2. Peel the bell pepper with a vegetable peeler and remove the seeds. Roughly cut. Finely slice the broccoli florets so there are no thick stems (the cooking time is very short and thick stems will stay hard).

3. Peel, smash, and finely chop the garlic. Peel and grate the ginger.

4. Prepare the add-ons. Roughly chop the macadamia nuts (if you can't find raw, you can also use roasted and salted). Slice the scallions. Have the coconut aminos, rice vinegar, water, and yacon syrup ready to use.

5. Heat a big skillet on medium heat, add 2 or 3 tablespoons (28 to 45 ml) of oil, and when hot, add the chicken without the marinade liquid (reserve it

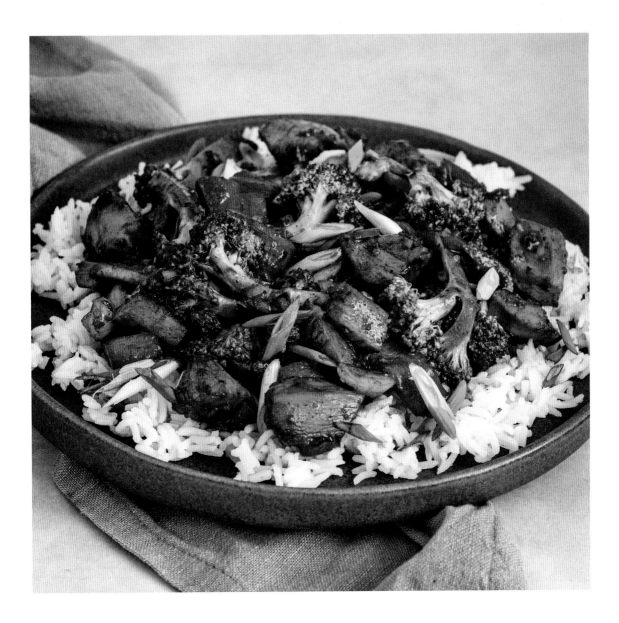

as you will use it later). Sear the chicken for about 7 minutes until golden brown. Take the chicken out and place into a clean bowl.

6. Add 1 or 2 more tablespoons (28 to 45 ml) of oil to the pan and add the bell pepper, broccoli, garlic, and ginger. Toss well and start adding small quantities of water so the garlic and ginger don't burn. Cook for about 4 minutes, stirring well. Add the reserved chicken marinade, coconut aminos,

rice vinegar, macadamia nuts, and chicken and toss well. Bring the mixture up to a boil and simmer for a few minutes. Then, add the scallions (keep some for garnish) and taste and add salt and pepper if necessary. Add the yacon syrup and take off the heat.

7. Serve on top of Indian basmati rice and garnish with fresh scallions. Add some Tabasco Red Pepper Sauce if you want a little bit of spice.

TURKEY MEATBALLS WITH SORGHUM SPAGHETTI AND PESTO

Who doesn't like meatballs? They are such a versatile and delicious food and can be made in big batches in advance and frozen. You can serve them with tortillas, in sandwiches, with salad, or as appetizers. One of my favorite ways to eat them is with sorghum spaghetti (or any lectin-free pasta) and pesto.

Preparation time:
25 minutes

Cooking time:
15 minutes

Makes:
40 meatballs

1 yellow onion

1 generous handful of fresh parsley

2 pounds (900 g) ground pasture-raised turkey

4 garlic cloves, minced

½ teaspoon dried basil

½ teaspoon dried oregano

1½ teaspoons salt

½ teaspoon freshly ground pepper

1 teaspoon paprika

2 pastured eggs

5 tablespoons (44 g) sorghum flour or (56 g) semolina flour ([44 g] cassava or [35 g] almond flour can also be used)

4 tablespoons (60 ml) extra-virgin olive oil

1. Preheat the oven to 400°F (200°C, or gas mark 6) and line a big baking tray with parchment paper.

2. Mince the onion and parsley in a food processor and add them to the ground turkey.

3. Add all the spices and eggs and combine well. Add the flour gradually until some of the moisture is absorbed. Don't worry if the mixture still seems a little wet. The meatballs will dry out when cooking.

4. Scoop about 1 tablespoon (15 ml) of the mixture and form small balls with your hands. Arrange on a baking tray covered with parchment paper.

5. Generously brush all the meatballs with olive oil.

6. Bake for about 13 minutes until no longer soft to the touch and finish on broil for a little color (2 to 3 minutes).

7. They can be eaten warm or cold. Use within 1 to 2 days. See sidebar for my favorite way of using them in a meal.

SERVING SUGGESTION:

To make one serving of Turkey Meatballs with Sorghum Spaghetti and Pesto, you need four cooked meatballs, sliced in half, about 4 tablespoons (60 g) of pesto, some extra-virgin olive oil, and one serving of lectin-free pasta. First, sear the meatballs, cut-side down, in a little bit of olive oil, just to warm them up. Add the boiled pasta with 2 tablespoons (28 ml) of the boiling water and the pesto. Warm and toss everything for 1 minute and serve. If you eat dairy, grate 1 tablespoon (5 g) of Parmigiano Reggiano on top. You can use any pesto from this book.

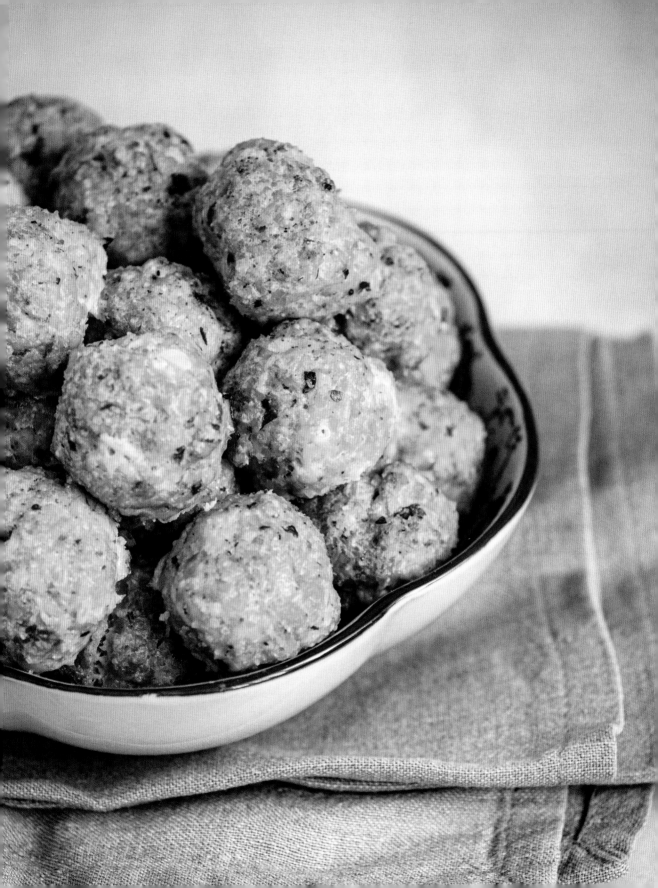

BAKED CHICKEN SATAY

Some can't imagine chicken satay without peanuts and soy. Well, not only it is possible, but this version is delicious, easy to make, and healthier than the original. You will have to start by making the No-Peanuts Satay Sauce from page 83. Even if the sauce will be served warm, you can make it one day in advance and warm it in the oven when the chicken is cooking. You don't even need a grill for cooking the chicken as the oven will work very well (but please feel free to use the grill if you want). I love to serve this as a main dish with boiled savoy cabbage or a big, green salad or as an appetizer for a small gathering.

Preparation time:
30 minutes

Cooking time:
15–20 minutes

Serves:
2–5

14 ounces (400 g) skinless, boneless pasture-raised chicken breast

2 shallots, cut into quarters

1 cup (256 g) No-Peanuts Satay Sauce (page 83)

FOR THE MARINADE:

½ cup (120 ml) full-fat coconut milk

3 tablespoons (45 ml) extra-virgin olive oil

3 big garlic cloves, grated or mashed

1 thumb-size piece of fresh ginger, grated

1 teaspoon ground coriander

1 teaspoon ground turmeric

1 teaspoon salt

Juice of ½ lime

½ teaspoon freshly ground pepper

FOR SERVING:

Fresh cilantro

Sea salt flakes

5–6 drops Tabasco Red Pepper Sauce, or more to taste

TOOLS:

Bamboo or wooden skewers, soaked in water for a few hours before use

1. Cut the chicken and portion it into thin strips. They don't all have to be the same length (that's not possible) but about the same thickness and width.

2. Make the marinade: Combine all the ingredients in a mixing bowl or a big glass container with a lid. Add the chicken strips to the marinade, mix well, cover the bowl or the container, and place in the fridge until you are ready to cook the chicken. For best results, try to marinate it for at least 2 hours. It can even be done overnight. Soak your bamboo skewers in water, the longer the better (so they don't burn).

3. About 40 minutes before mealtime, preheat the oven to 400°F (200°C, or gas mark 6), or use the grill setting on 425°F (220°C, or gas mark 7) if you have that.

4. Take the chicken out of the fridge, skewer the strips onto the bamboo or wooden skewers, and arrange them on a baking sheet. Add the quartered shallots to the pan.

5. Bake for about 20 minutes until cooked through on a normal baking setting or for about 15 minutes on the grill setting. About halfway through, you can flip them.

6. Meanwhile, add the satay sauce to an ovenproof serving dish and insert it in the oven for a few minutes to get warm.

7. When the chicken is ready, arrange the skewers on the serving dish on top of the warm satay sauce. Garnish with fresh cilantro, pepper, sea salt flakes, and Tabasco Red Pepper Sauce, if you want, and the roasted shallots.

CHICKEN-TAHINI SALAD WITH CHICKPEAS AND ASPARAGUS

This recipe is perfect for when you have some leftover chicken. I always keep pressure cooked chickpeas in the freezer, but you can also use chickpeas from a can. It's such an easy salad to make, but the combination is both delicious and nutritious. You can eat it any time of the day and easily make it on rotation for your weekly menu by having cooked chicken and chickpeas ready to use. You can add a big, green salad next to it or serve it with the Sorghum Morning Bread Rolls (page 60) or romaine boats.

Preparation time:
20 minutes

Cooking time:
10 minutes

Serves:
2–3

FOR THE TAHINI SAUCE (makes about ½ cup [120 g]):

3 heaping tablespoons (45 g) tahini

Zest of 1 organic lemon

Juice of ½ lemon

3 tablespoons (45 ml) extra-virgin olive oil

1 teaspoon capers, rinsed

6 tablespoons (90 ml) water

Pinch of salt

Pinch of freshly ground pepper

Pinch of ground ginger

½ teaspoon local or raw honey or yacon syrup

FOR THE SALAD:

1 bunch asparagus (seasoned with salt, freshly ground pepper, and extra-virgin olive oil)

2 tablespoons (16 g) sesame seeds

1 cup (225 g) shredded, cooked or leftover chicken

1 cup (164 g) pressure cooked chickpeas, or [240 g] canned chickpeas, drained and rinsed

2 tablespoons (28 ml) extra-virgin olive oil

1 heaping tablespoon (15 g) tahini dressing, or more to taste

1 tablespoon (3 g) fresh chives, chopped (or 1 teaspoon dried chives)

Juice of ½ lemon, or more to taste

Salt and freshly ground pepper to taste (start with ¼ teaspoon of each)

Optional: add a few drops of Tabasco Red Pepper Sauce or another compliant hot sauce

1. Make the sauce in advance by adding all the ingredients to a blender and combine until creamy.

2. Roast the asparagus in the oven for 10 minutes at 400°F (200°C, or gas mark 6), with salt, pepper, and a drizzle of olive oil. Let it cool down and chop. Alternatively, if it's easier for you, you can steam it or sauté it in a pan or even use it raw.

3. Lightly toast the sesame seeds in a pan.

4. Add all the salad ingredients to a mixing bowl. Combine, taste, and adjust the seasoning to your preference.

TURKEY BURGER WITH DUKKAH SPICE MIX AND PESTO

A burger requires a little bit of planning, but even so, this one is so easy to make that you will probably make it on a weekly basis. You need a jar of pesto, a jar of marinated onions (which can be made even 1 hour before), and burger buns or a low-carb option, like lettuce leaves. Olive paste is easy to find in health food stores or online, and if not, you can use chopped olives or make your own tapenade with the help of a food processor. The star of this show is the Dukkah Spice and Nut Mix, made of ground hazelnuts, sesame seeds, black cumin seeds, coriander seeds, cumin seeds, black peppercorns, and sea salt. You will find the recipe on page 28. Not only does it give an amazing depth of taste, but it also helps with the texture. This quantity makes five patties, and the recipe is for four burgers. Enjoy the one patty left over for breakfast the next day.

Preparation:
45 minutes

Cooking time:
10 minutes

Serves:
4

FOR THE BURGER PATTIES (makes 5 patties):

1 pound (455 g) ground pasture-raised turkey

4 tablespoons (32 g) Dukkah Spice and Nut Mix (page 28)

2 tablespoons (8 g) finely chopped parsley

Pinch of garlic powder

Pinch of onion powder

½ teaspoon salt

Extra-virgin olive oil for cooking (to coat the pan)

FOR THE MARINATED ONIONS:

1 red onion, finely sliced into rings, with a mandolin

6 tablespoons (90 ml) extra-virgin olive oil, or more if necessary to cover the onions

2 tablespoons (28 ml) apple cider vinegar

FOR ASSEMBLING THE BURGERS (makes 4 burgers):

5 tablespoons (75 g) pesto (I recommend the Bitter Greens Pesto, page 92)

4 Hamburger Buns (page 52) or lettuce leaves for a low-carb bun replacement

2 handfuls of arugula leaves

3 tablespoons (75 g) olive paste

Marinated red onions and liquid

More Dukkah Spice and Nut Mix for garnish

---

1. To make the burger patties: Mix all the ingredients together, form five patties, gently flatten them, and cook them in a little bit of olive or avocado oil in a cast-iron pan or a nonstick pan. It will take about 5 minutes per side on medium heat until the patties are cooked through and reach an internal temperature of 165°F (74°C).

2. To make the marinated onions: You can make these in advance, even a day before. Add the sliced onions to a jar, top with olive oil and apple cider vinegar, cover, and shake well. Shake occasionally.

3. To assemble the burgers: Spread pesto on the bun, top with the arugula leaves, add the burger patties, top with olive paste, and generously top with onions. Sprinkle with Dukkah Spice and Nut Mix and drizzle with the liquid from the onions.

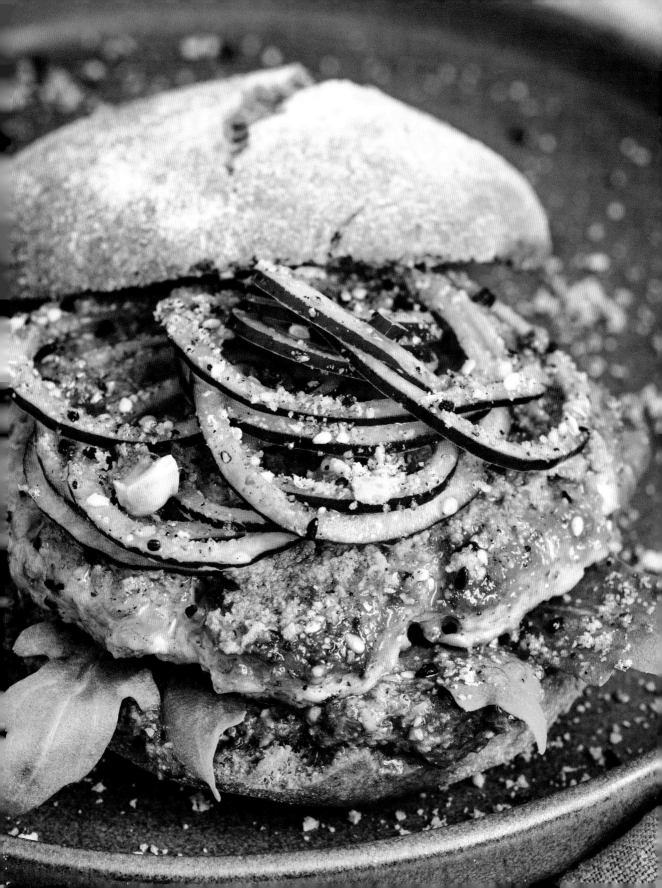

CHICKEN GYRO PLATTER WITH TZATZIKI SAUCE

If you would ask me what type of food I want to eat for the rest of my life, something like this would be the answer. I love Greek food. I created this meal after a series of trips to a Greek restaurant where my husband would order the Chicken Gyro Platter and I would watch him eating. I decided I wanted to create my own version that I can enjoy at home anytime I want. It's better to plan this meal in advance and make sure you have the pita breads already made so you don't have to spend too much time in the kitchen. This is a great family dinner for sharing and even a family cooking project, where everyone can be in charge of one element of the dish.

Preparation time:
1 hour

Cooking time:
20 minutes

Serves:
4

FOR THE CHICKEN MARINADE (make in advance):

½ cup (115 g) full-fat goat, sheep, or buffalo yogurt

1 teaspoon ground coriander

½ teaspoon cumin

2 teaspoons oregano

1 heaping teaspoon paprika

2 teaspoons minced garlic

¼ teaspoon freshly ground pepper

1 teaspoon salt

Zest of 1 organic lemon

2 tablespoons (28 ml) fresh lemon juice

FOR THE CHICKEN:

1⅓ pounds (600 g) boneless, skinless chicken thighs

3–4 tablespoons (45 to 60 ml) extra-virgin olive oil

FOR THE TZATZIKI SAUCE:

½ cup (115 g) full-fat goat, sheep, or buffalo yogurt

½ cup (70 g) peeled, deseeded, and chopped cucumber

2 tablespoons (28 ml) fresh lemon juice

1 heaping (4 g) tablespoon finely chopped dill

1 heaping (4 g) tablespoon finely chopped parsley

FOR THE FRIES:

2 medium sweet potatoes (use more if everyone loves them)

1½ tablespoons (25 ml) extra-virgin olive oil

Pinch of salt

FOR SERVING:

4 lectin-free pita breads (It's best to use the Multi-Purpose Dough from page 52 but Easy Cassava Flour Tortillas from page 58 would work too.)

Any green salad or sprouts you have and/or shredded cabbage

TO MAKE THE MARINADE:

Make the marinade in advance, about 2 hours before you start, or you can make it in the morning or whenever you have time during the day. In a bowl, combine the yogurt with all the spices, the lemon zest, and lemon juice, then add the chicken, and mix well. Put everything in a silicon bag or a glass container, make sure the chicken is covered in the marinade, cover well, and put in the fridge until the cooking time. It will be great if you can marinate for at least 2 hours.

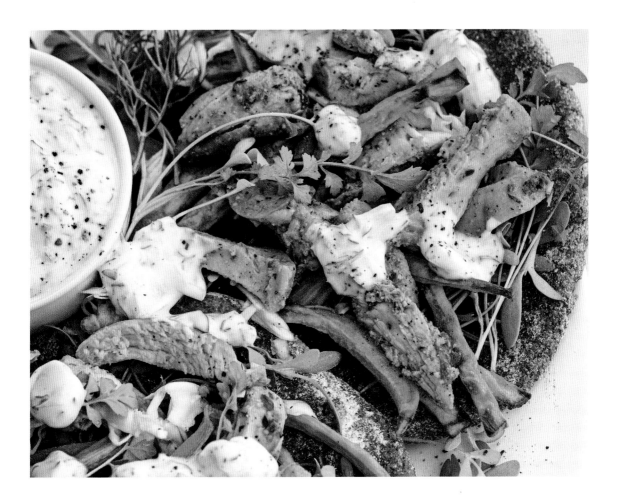

TO COOK THE CHICKEN:

Heat 3 to 4 tablespoons (45 to 60 ml) of olive oil in a big skillet. Add the chicken with the marinade and cook for about 10 minutes on each side (time will also depend on how the chicken is cut or how big the pieces are). The chicken should be cooked through and reach an internal temperature of 165°F (74°C). Chicken thighs are forgiving and will not dry out like chicken breast but keep an eye on them.

TO MAKE THE FRIES:

Peel the sweet potatoes, wash with cold water and dry. Cut off the round ends and slice lengthwise. Cut the slices again into evenly sized sticks. Add to a baking sheet, drizzle with just a tiny bit of olive oil, toss to coat them with the oil, and arrange them so they are not crowded in the pan. Cook at 375°F (190°C, or gas mark 5) without touching for about 20 minutes, but it will depend on how thick the fries are (keep an eye on them so they don't burn). When they are ready, remove them from the oven, stir with a spatula, and let set on the hot pan until the rest of the food is ready. Generously season with salt just before serving (salt will turn them mushy during cooking).

TO MAKE THE TZATZIKI SAUCE:

Combine all the ingredients. This can be made in advance and kept in a glass jar in the fridge for up to 12 hours.

TO SERVE:

Add the pita breads on a platter with the chicken, fries, tzatziki sauce, any green salad you have, and/or shredded cabbage.

BISTRO SALAD BOWL WITH CHICKEN AND ASPARAGUS

Don't get fooled by the word "salad." This is a complete and satisfying main dish, and you can eat it anytime of the day. The good news is, it will be good even cold, so it will make a great lunchbox meal.

Preparation time:
20 minutes

Cooking time:
20 minutes

Serves:
4

FOR THE CHICKEN AND ASPARAGUS:

2 big chicken breasts (4½ to 5½ ounces [125 to 150 g] each), boneless and skinless

¼ teaspoon salt

¼ teaspoon freshly ground pepper

2–3 tablespoons (28 to 45 ml) extra-virgin olive oil

2–3 sprigs fresh rosemary

2 garlic cloves, smashed

½ teaspoon paprika

1 bunch asparagus, woody ends trimmed

Salt and freshly ground pepper for finishing

FOR THE SALAD:

4 generous handfuls of green or bistro salad mix

2–3 red radishes, finely sliced

1 avocado, cubed

2 hard-boiled pastured eggs, sliced into wedges

1 small handful of caper berries, finely sliced

FOR THE DRESSING:

1 teaspoon Dijon mustard

4 tablespoons (60 ml) extra-virgin olive oil

1 tablespoon (15 ml) aged balsamic vinegar

Salt and freshly ground pepper to taste

1. Rub the chicken breasts with salt and pepper.

2. Add the olive oil to a skillet on medium heat. When hot, add the chicken breast, rosemary sprigs, and garlic and cook for about 10 minutes on the first side. Flip the chicken on the second side and sprinkle paprika on top (paprika tends to burn and become bitter, which is why I prefer to add it at the end of the cooking process). Cook for 5 more minutes.

3. Push the chicken to the side and add the asparagus to the same pan. Cook al dente for about 3 minutes, stirring occasionally. Don't overcook the asparagus. At this point, both the chicken and the asparagus should be ready. Slice the chicken breast and check that it is cooked through and no longer pink in the middle. You also don't want to overcook it, as it will become tough. Place the chicken and asparagus onto a cutting board and let rest for 5 minutes.

4. While the chicken is cooking, you can prepare the rest of the ingredients. Make the mustard vinaigrette by whisking all the ingredients together until emulsified.

5. Split the salad mix into four serving bowls and top with radishes, avocado, and egg wedges.

6. Slice the chicken and add on top of each bowl. Also add the asparagus.

7. Top with the caper berries and mustard vinaigrette. Mix and serve, as a main dish.

MOROCCAN-STYLE CHICKEN AND VEGETABLE STEW

I love spice mixes, as they make the cooking process faster and easier. *Ras el hanout*, which literally means *top of the shelf spices*, is a Moroccan spice mix you can find anywhere in the world. It works beautifully with chicken, beef, or lamb. This stew is made in a pressure cooker and can be served with Indian basmati rice, or millet, or if you want to keep it low carb, with a big, green salad or Cabbage Salad with Dill (page 102).

Preparation time:
30 minutes

Cooking time:
45 minutes

Serves:
4

2 big onions, sliced or roughly chopped

2 medium tomatoes, peeled and deseeded, cut into big chunks

2 medium carrots, whole

1 medium parsnip, whole

1 big zucchini, peeled and deseeded, cut into big chunks

½ cup of chickpeas ([120 g] canned or [82 g] pressure cooked)

½ small head cabbage, cut into large wedges

4 tablespoons (60 ml) extra-virgin olive oil

1⅓ pounds (600 g) chicken with bones
(about 6 chicken thighs)

2 heaping teaspoons ras el hanout spice mix

1 teaspoon salt

½ teaspoon freshly ground pepper

2½ cups (570 ml) water

2 teaspoons tapioca flour dissolved in 4 tablespoons (60 ml) cold water

FOR SERVING:

More salt to taste

2–3 cups (348 to 522 g) cooked millet or (318 to 474 g) Indian basmati rice

Fresh parsley and/or cilantro

1. Prepare all the vegetables.

2. Heat the olive oil in the pressure cooker on medium heat or use the sauté option if available.

3. Add the onions and cook for a few minutes until the onions soften up and become fragrant.

4. Add the chicken, skin-side down, making space in between the onions. Let the chicken brown on one side and then turn on the second side. It will take about 10 minutes in total. Stir if the onions are starting to get stuck to the pan.

5. Add the spices and the roughly chopped tomatoes. Stir well so the spice mix is coating everything in the pan. Cook for about 2 minutes and add a few tablespoons (45 to 60 ml) of water to deglaze the pan so the spices don't burn.

6. Add all the vegetables in layers, starting with the carrots, parsnip, zucchini, chickpeas, and cabbage. The cabbage should be on top.

7. Add the water, cover, and start your pressure cooker. Set to cook on high pressure (or the meat option if available) for 10 minutes. Allow the pressure to release naturally.

8. After removing the lid, start the heat on low and add the tapioca flour and water mixture. Stir and simmer for a few minutes. Taste and add more salt if necessary.

9. Serve with millet or pressure cooked and cooled Indian basmati rice. Garnish with fresh parsley and cilantro.

YELLOW CHICKEN CURRY WITH CAULIFLOWER RICE

When my husband and I used to eat out a lot, one of our favorite dishes was yellow chicken curry with rice. The restaurant Wagamama shared a similar recipe during the pandemic on their social media channels. I wanted to re-create something similar that is also clean and free of soy sauce or other questionable bottled ingredients. Coconut aminos came to the rescue. Cauliflower rice is absolutely delicious in this combination, and my husband, who is not on any diet and can eat whatever he wants, loved this dish. You can stretch this meal to four servings (maybe if small kids are eating), but for hungry adults, I would say this makes for two generous servings.

Preparation time:
15 minutes

Cooking time:
30 minutes

Serves:
2–4

FOR THE CURRY SAUCE:

2 medium onions, chopped

2 tablespoons (28 ml) extra-virgin olive oil

1 thumb-size piece of fresh ginger, grated

4 garlic cloves, minced

2 teaspoons curry powder

1 teaspoon ground turmeric

1 cup (235 ml) chicken or vegetable stock

3 teaspoons (8 g) tapioca flour

2 tablespoons (28 ml) coconut aminos

½ teaspoon salt

Freshly ground pepper

½ cup (120 ml) full-fat coconut milk

FOR THE CHICKEN:

4 chicken thighs, with or without bones

½ teaspoon salt

Freshly ground pepper

2 tablespoons (28 ml) extra-virgin olive, (28 ml) avocado, or (28 g) coconut oil

FOR THE CAULIFLOWER RICE:

2 carrots, chopped into big cubes

2 tablespoons (28 ml) coconut aminos

1 pound (455 g) cauliflower rice

FOR SERVING:

Green salad leaves

TO PREPARE THE SAUCE:
You can make this sauce in advance and reheat. Sauté the onions in a saucepan with the olive oil. When they are translucent and fragrant, add the ginger and garlic. Stir well and cook for 2 more minutes, continuing to stir. Add the curry powder and turmeric, again stirring well. Add a few tablespoons (45 to 60 ml) of vegetable stock so the spices won't burn. Add the tapioca flour straight to the saucepan, stir well, and then add the vegetable or chicken stock. Continue with the coconut aminos, salt, and pepper and cook on low heat until it reaches the boiling point and starts thickening, about 5 minutes. Use a whisk to get a smooth texture. Start adding the coconut milk, stirring well. Cook for a few more minutes. The texture should be soft and creamy.

TO PREPARE THE CHICKEN AND CAULIFLOWER RICE:
Season the chicken with salt and pepper and fry skin-side down in the oil on medium heat. It will take about 15 to 20 minutes. Halfway through, flip the chicken over to the other side, When the chicken is golden on both sides, take it out

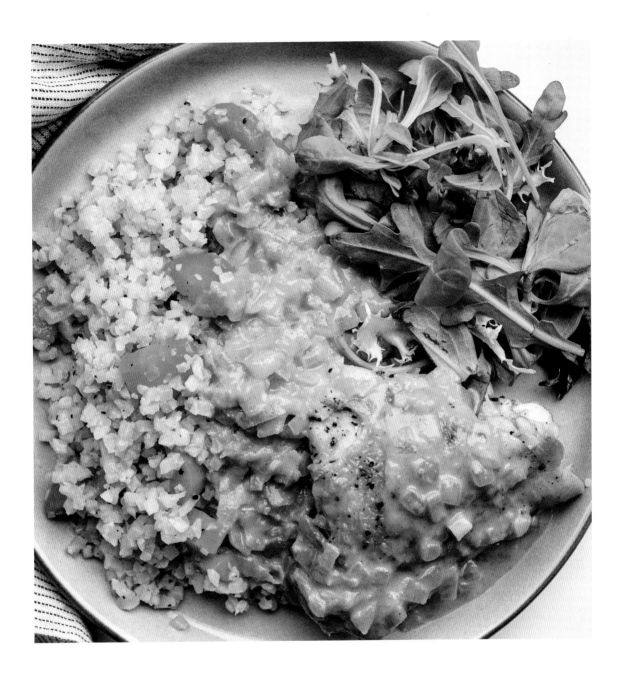

of the skillet. Add the carrots to the same pan and sauté for about 5 minutes. Add the coconut aminos, stir well, and cook for 1 more minute. Add the cauliflower rice, stir well, and cook for a few minutes until it starts to soften up but retains the texture. Add the chicken back to the pan, cover, and cook for a couple of minutes until the chicken is cooked through.

TO SERVE:
Add the chicken and cauliflower rice to a serving plate and top with the yellow curry. Serve with green salad leaves.

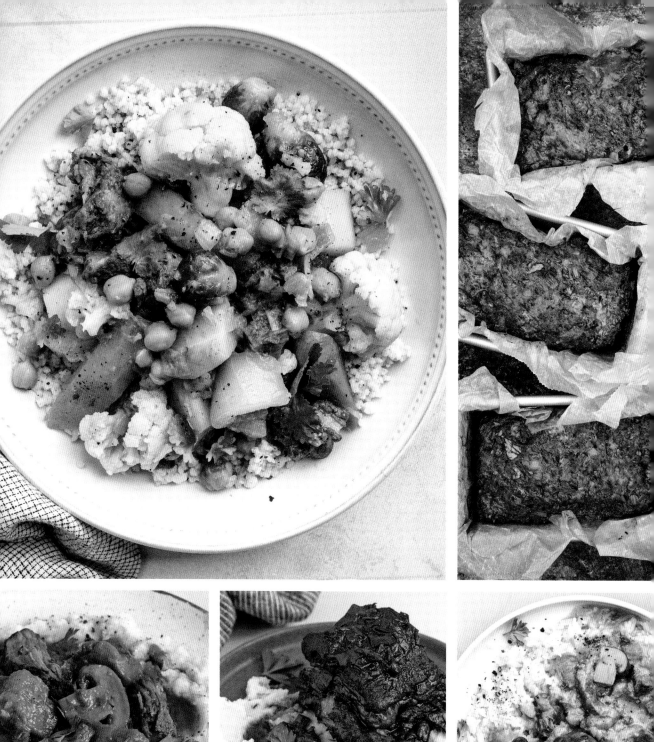
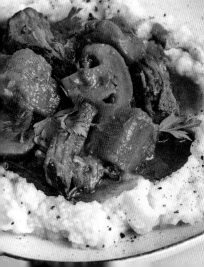
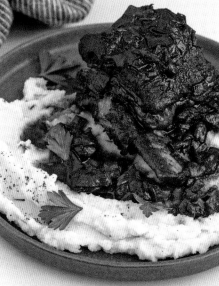
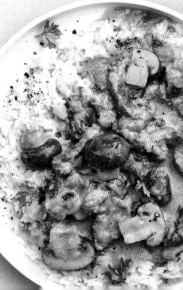

10

Main Courses with Beef, Lamb, or Pork

Clockwise from top left: Moroccan-Style Lamb and Vegetable Stew and Millet (page 146); Chunky Italian Sausage Meat Loaf (page 140); Creamy but Dairy-Free Beef Stroganoff (page 142); Five-Spice Beef Ribs with Parsnip and Celeriac Purée (page 148); Pulled Beef and Gravy with Cauliflower-Parsnip Purée (page 144)

CHUNKY ITALIAN SAUSAGE MEAT LOAF

This meat loaf tastes like Italian sausage, thanks to the combination of spices. This is made with beef, but you can certainly make it with ground chicken. I love making meat loaf because we slice and freeze the leftovers, and we have a few more meals just ready to thaw. You can serve two chunky slices of meat loaf with a big green salad, my favorite way, or with some steamed vegetables, like broccoli and asparagus.

Preparation time:
30 minutes

Cooking time:
45 minutes–
1 hour

Serves:
6–8

2 roasted red bell peppers (½ cup [90 g]), peeled and deseeded, finely chopped, divided

FOR THE GLAZE (optional):

¼ cup (45 g) roasted red bell peppers, chopped

1 tablespoon (15 ml) apple cider vinegar

1 tablespoon (15 ml) extra-virgin olive oil

Pinch of salt and freshly ground pepper

FOR THE MEAT LOAF:

3 tablespoons (45 ml) extra-virgin olive oil (to generously cover the pan)

1 small fennel bulb, finely chopped

1 big leek (mostly the white part), finely chopped

2 sprigs thyme

½ teaspoon dried oregano

½ teaspoon fennel seeds

1 teaspoon paprika

½ teaspoon ground coriander

⅛ (28 ml) cup water

1 pound 2 ounces (500 g) grass-fed ground beef

¼ cup (45 g) roasted red bell peppers, chopped

½ teaspoon thick sweet potato purée

4 garlic cloves, minced

1 tablespoon (15 ml) apple cider vinegar

1 pastured egg

¼ cup (12 g) chopped fresh chives

¼ cup (16 g) chopped fresh dill

½ cup (30 g) chopped fresh parsley

1 ½ teaspoon salt, divided

¾ teaspoon freshly ground pepper, divided

3 tablespoons (27 g) sorghum flour (or cassava flour)

FOR SERVING:

Big green salad

---

1. Heat the olive oil in a big skillet and sauté the fennel and leeks until golden brown, soft, and fragrant. Stir occasionally.

2. Add 1 teaspoon salt, ½ teaspoon freshly ground pepper, and the spices and stir for a few minutes until the spices release their oils and flavors. Don't let them burn. When they start sticking to the pan, add about ⅛ cup (28 ml) of water to deglaze the pan. Give it a last stir and cook for 1 more minute.

3. Preheat the oven to 350°F (180°C, or gas mark 4) and prepare a loaf pan or three mini loaf pans.

4. In a big bowl, mix the ground beef with the sautéed vegetables, ¼ cup (45 g) of roasted red peppers, the sweet potato purée, garlic, apple cider vinegar, egg, and fresh herbs. Add ½ teaspoon salt and ¼ teaspoon pepper. Mix well.

5. Add the flour and mix again. If it looks too wet, add more flour, but make sure the mixture remains moist. The quantity of flour might depend on how watery your sweet potato is (a thick, baked mashed sweet potato will need less flour than a watery, canned sweet potato purée).

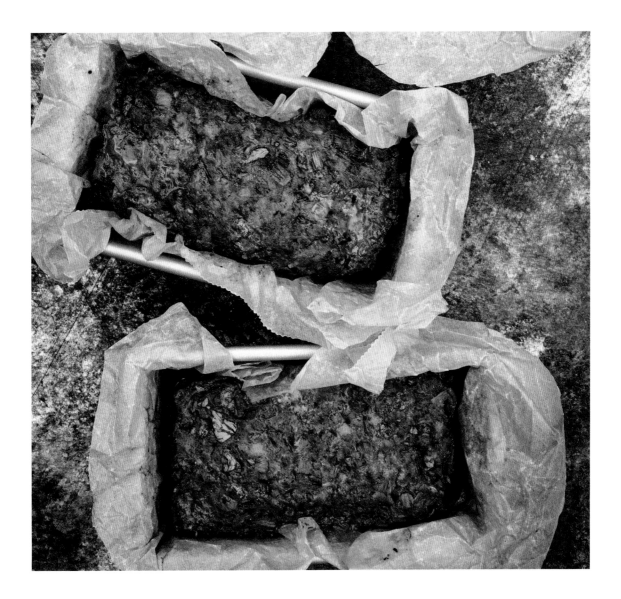

6. Place the mixture into the prepared loaf pan or distribute the mixture between the three mini loaf pans if using. Level well, making sure there is no air left inside the meat loafs.

7. Bake for about 1 hour for one large meat loaf or 45 minutes for three mini meat loafs until the meat loafs are no longer soft to the touch, start browning on top, and reach an internal temperature of 160°F (71°C).

8. While the meat loaf is baking, you can make the optional roasted red pepper glaze. Mix all the glaze ingredients in a blender.

9. When the meat loaf is ready, remove from the oven and let slightly cool down. Remove from the loaf pan, brush with the glaze if using, and serve with a big green salad.

10. The meat loaf can be frozen whole or sliced and reheated in the oven.

CREAMY BUT DAIRY-FREE BEEF STROGANOFF

Beef Stroganoff needs no introduction. I think everyone has eaten it at least once in their life. This recipe doesn't exactly follow the original instructions. It's dairy-free and made in a pressure cooker. But it's creamy and delicious, without the use of sour cream. While the original recipe requires a tender cut of meat, like top sirloin or beef tenderloin, since you are using a pressure cooker, you can use tougher cuts of meat here. Just adjust the cooking time accordingly. Serve with lectin-free pasta, pressure cooked and cooled Indian basmati rice, or Cauliflower and Root Vegetable Purée with Turmeric and Chives (page 168).

Preparation time:
20 minutes

Cooking time:
35 minutes

Serves:
2

3–4 tablespoons (45 to 60 ml) extra-virgin olive oil

3 medium yellow onions, chopped

1 pound (455 g) beef, cut into bite-size, thin strips (preferably tender cuts of meat, like top sirloin)

About 10 medium brown mushrooms, cut into halves or if bigger, in quarters

3 big garlic cloves, smashed and finely chopped

Leaves of 3 sprigs thyme

1 cup (235 ml) water or stock

1½ teaspoons salt, or more to taste

½ teaspoon freshly ground pepper, plus more for finishing

½ cup (120 ml) hemp milk, homemade (page 33) or store-bought

2 teaspoons tapioca flour

1 bunch parsley, chopped

FOR SERVING:

Pressure cooked and cooled (reheated) Indian basmati rice or root vegetable mash

Steamed broccoli, boiled cabbage, or a simple cabbage salad

1. Start the pressure cooker on medium heat or use the sauté option if available. Add olive oil to generously cover the bottom.

2. Add the chopped onions and sauté for about 10 minutes, stirring often, until the onions are golden and fragrant.

3. Add the beef, stir well, and cook for about 5 minutes on medium-to-high heat, stirring often.

4. Add the mushrooms and stir well. Add the garlic and thyme, stir, and let everything cook for about 5 more minutes until the mushrooms release their flavor.

5. Add the water or stock and salt and pepper, cover, and set the pressure cooker to 15 to 20 minutes, depending on the cut of your meat (a tender cut will need 15 minutes, a tougher cut a little more). When the time is done, let the pressure release naturally.

6. Dissolve the tapioca flour in ½ cup (120 ml) of cold hemp milk.

7. When the pressure is released, remove the lid, start the heat again, and add the tapioca flour and hemp milk mixture. Stir well and simmer for 5 more minutes. Add fresh parsley before serving.

8. Serve on pressure cooked and cooled (reheated) Indian basmati rice or root vegetable mash with steamed broccoli, boiled cabbage, or a simple cabbage salad.

PORK PAPRIKASH

With my Eastern European roots, I can't think of a better comfort dish than a hearty stew or paprikash. This is one of the few recipes I like to add white potatoes to, but if you are not ready for them, simply use Japanese sweet potatoes (those with white flesh). To remove lectins in white potatoes, I cook them first in a pressure cooker and add them to the dish 10 minutes before it's ready. It's very important you buy the best quality of paprika you can get, as that could make or break this dish. You would be surprised how much bad-quality paprika is on the market.

Preparation time:
30 minutes

Cooking time:
1 hour 30 minutes

Serves:
6

Lard or extra-virgin olive oil (to generously cover the pan)

7 medium yellow onions, chopped

2 pounds (900 g) pork leg cut (ham) or tenderloin, cut into bite-size pieces or a little bigger

2 teaspoons salt

¼ teaspoon freshly ground pepper

6 garlic cloves, minced

¼ teaspoon ground coriander

3 heaping (21 g) teaspoons sweet Hungarian paprika

Optional: If you want the stew to be spicy, add extra spicy paprika or cayenne.

1 sprig fresh thyme

1 sprig fresh rosemary

Optional: if you don't have fresh spices, you can add dried spices or replace with herbs de Provence mix, about 1 teaspoon.

1 big carrot, chopped

1 parsnip, chopped

1 small celeriac (celery root), chopped

About 2½ cups (570 ml) hot water

3–4 pressure cooked and cooled white potatoes, peeled and cut into big chunks

1 bunch fresh parsley, chopped

1. Add the fat to a heated big heavy pot, like a cast iron, French, or Dutch oven, with a lid.

2. Add the chopped onions and sauté for about 10 to 15 minutes on low heat until the onions become translucent, fragrant, and soft but remain white. Stir occasionally.

3. Add the pork pieces to the pot and cook, stirring often, for about 10 minutes. Add the spices. Stir well so all the meat gets coated with the spices (the heat will remain on low or somewhere in between medium and the lowest setting). Nothing should stick to the pan, as paprika becomes bitter and loses its vibrant color if burnt. Add a few tablespoons (45 to 60 ml) of water, cover, and simmer on low heat for about 10 minutes.

4. Take the lid off and add the carrots, parsnip, and celeriac. Add about 2 cups (475 ml) of hot water, stir well, and cover with the lid. Let simmer on low heat for about 45 minutes. Open and stir occasionally and add more water if necessary (again, it should not stick to the pan).

5. Add the already cooked potatoes, combine so everything gets coated with the sauce, cover, and simmer for 10 more minutes.

6. Add fresh parsley, taste, and adjust for salt if necessary.

PULLED BEEF AND GRAVY WITH CAULIFLOWER-PARSNIP PURÉE

Melt-in-your-mouth beef in a rich, delicious sauce, served with a purée, is a comforting meal for the entire family. However, this process can take hours, unless you use a pressure cooker. You can use a tougher cut of meat, like a beef round, that will be perfectly cooked in 1 hour. Don't get overwhelmed by the long cooking time, as a lot of it is passive time, and you can prepare other things while the pressure cooker does the work. Make sure you bring the meat to room temperature before cooking.

Preparation time:
30 minutes

Cooking time:
1 hour 30 minutes

Serves:
4

FOR THE BEEF:

2¼ pounds (1 kg) beef round

1 teaspoon salt

3 big carrots

2 big parsnips

3 celery ribs

3 medium onions

½ fennel bulb (if small, use 1 whole bulb)

5 garlic cloves

3–4 tablespoons (45 to 60 ml) extra-virgin olive oil

4–6 medium mushrooms (button)

1 teaspoon fresh thyme leaves or ¼ teaspoon dried

1 teaspoon fresh rosemary or ¼ teaspoon dried

1 teaspoon fresh oregano or ¼ teaspoon dried

1 teaspoon paprika

2 bay leaves

½ teaspoon salt

½ teaspoon freshly ground pepper

1 tablespoon (15 ml) aged balsamic vinegar

1 tablespoon (15 ml) coconut aminos

2 cups (475 ml) hot vegetable stock or water

1 to 2 teaspoons tapioca flour dissolved in a few teaspoons (15 to 20 ml) water

FOR THE PURÉE:

1 medium cauliflower, florets

2 medium parsnips

1 teaspoon salt

1 tablespoon (15 ml) apple cider vinegar

Optional: 1 tablespoon (14 g) grass-fed butter

¼ teaspoon ground mustard

Salt and freshly ground pepper to taste

---

1. Take the beef out of the fridge 1 hour before cooking. Rinse, pat dry, and generously season with salt.

2. Prepare the vegetables and spices. Cut the carrots, parsnips, and celery into big chunks. Slice the onions and fennel into thin wedges. Peel and smash the garlic. Clean and halve the mushrooms.

3. Heat the olive oil in your pressure cooker on medium heat or use the sauté option if available.

4. Brown the beef on all sides. Add the onions and garlic and continue to sauté, stirring well so the vegetables get coated with oil and juices. Continue to cook until the onions and garlic become fragrant, 5 to 10 minutes. Add all the spices and herbs and the rest of the vegetables. Stir well and continue for 5 more minutes.

5. Add the balsamic vinegar and coconut aminos, stir well, and then add the stock or water.

6. Cover the pot and set the pressure cooker to 1 hour.

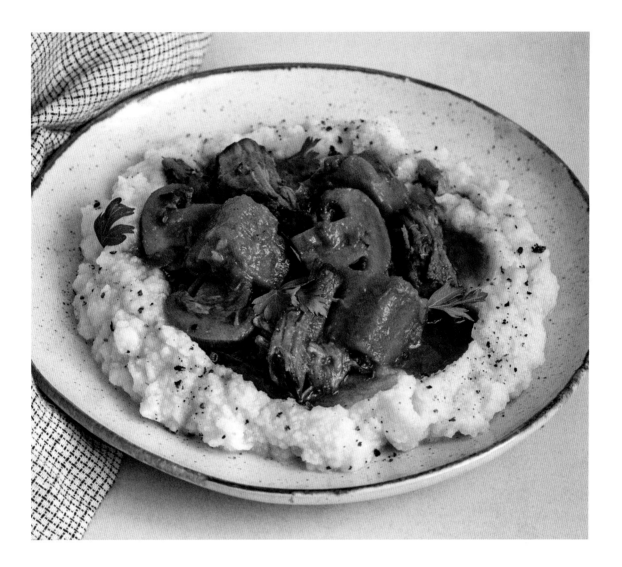

7. While the beef is cooking, prepare the cauliflower and parsnips. Boil them with salt and apple cider vinegar until fork-tender. Drain the liquid, saving ½ cup (60 ml) in case you need more liquid for blending. Blend, add the butter, and season with ground mustard and salt and pepper. When the beef is ready, you can rewarm it.

8. When the time for the beef has concluded, let the pressure release naturally for about 10 to 15 minutes. Place the meat and chunks of carrots, parsnips, and mushrooms onto a platter. Strain the liquid, pressing down on the vegetables to get all the juices out.

9. Put the liquid back on the heat and simmer for about 10 minutes. Add the tapioca flour and water mixture to the gravy. Simmer for a couple of minutes until it thickens.

10. Shred the meat and add it to the gravy together with the saved vegetables and cook for a couple of minutes until the meat warms up. Remove the bay leaves.

11. Serve the meat and vegetables on a bed of cauliflower and parsnip purée, garnished with fresh parsley. Serve with pickles or a fresh green salad.

MOROCCAN-STYLE LAMB AND VEGETABLE STEW WITH MILLET

I absolutely love Moroccan flavors, and couscous-style meals are some of my favorites. I actually had the chance to see a Moroccan mom preparing couscous from scratch, and the visual with the process stuck with me. She was also using a pressure cooker. It's hard to give you an exact preparation time and cooking time because it's done in one pot, and the process involves both active and passive times, but I can tell you it's an easy dish to make. Add more meat and vegetables if your family is really hungry and eats more animal protein, or more chickpeas and vegetables if you want to keep protein low. To make things easier, prepare the millet one day in advance.

Preparation time:
30 minutes

Cooking time:
1 hour

Serves:
2–4

1⅓ pounds (500 g) lamb neck

1 teaspoon ras el hanout spice mix

2 teaspoons salt, divided

¾ teaspoon freshly ground pepper, divided

3 big red onions, or a mix of red and yellow

3–4 tablespoons (45 to 60 ml) extra-virgin olive oil (to generously cover the bottom of the pot)

¼ cup (45 g) roasted red peppers, peeled and deseeded

1 tablespoon (15 ml) apple cider vinegar

1½ cups (355 ml) warm/hot water

1 big zucchini, peeled and deseeded

1 big parsnip

2 medium carrots

6 big cauliflower florets

10 Brussels sprouts

⅔ cup (160 g) canned chickpeas

1 small handful of fresh cilantro

1 small handful of fresh parsley

2–3 cups (348 to 522 g) cooked millet

1. Cut the lamb neck into bite-size cubes, trimming any big fatty parts.

2. Sprinkle the ras el hanout, 1 teaspoon salt, and ½ teaspoon pepper on top of the lamb and start massaging it into the meat.

3. Chop the onions.

4. Start your pressure cooker on medium heat or use the sauté option if available and generously coat the pan with olive oil. When the oil is hot, add the onions and sauté for about 7 to 10 minutes, stirring occasionally, or until the onions are fragrant and golden (don't let them get browned).

5. Add the meat, toss well, and cook for 10 more minutes, stirring every 2 minutes or so, so the spices don't get burnt. If you feel it sticking to the pan, either lower the heat or add a little bit of water. Add the roasted red peppers.

6. Add the apple cider vinegar and water, cover the pot, and pressure cook on high pressure for 15 minutes. When the time is up, let the pressure release naturally for 10 minutes and then release manually if there is anything left.

7. While the meat is cooking, prepare the veggies. Peel the zucchini and scoop out the seeds. Peel the parsnip and the carrot if you want (usually organic carrots can be left unpeeled; however, they'll look prettier if they are peeled). Cut the cauliflower into big florets and trim the ends of the Brussels sprouts. They should all be cut into big chunks, about 1 inch (2.5 cm) thick. Leave the Brussels

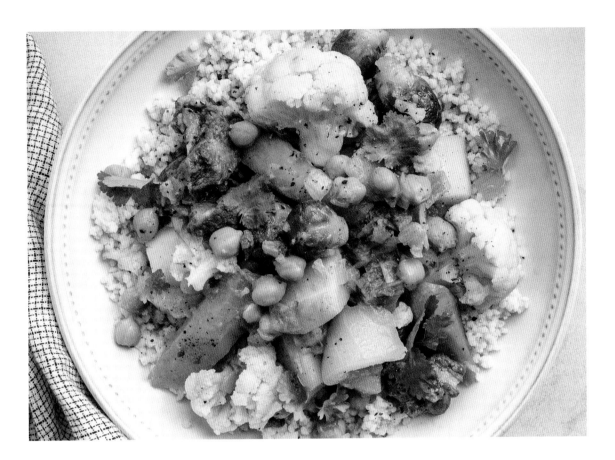

sprouts whole. Alternatively, you can use big wedges of white cabbage. Rinse the chickpeas.

8. By the time you are done with the veggies, the pressure should be released. Open the lid and add all the veggies on top along with 1 teaspoon salt and ¼ teaspoon pepper. Just gently toss so a little bit of the liquid coats them. They won't be immersed in liquid. Close the lid and set the pressure to 3 minutes. After the time is up, let the pressure release naturally for about 7 minutes and then release manually what's left.

9. Taste and add more salt if necessary. Just before ready to serve, add the fresh cilantro and parsley.

10. Serve the meat, vegetables, and sauce on top of cooked millet. The millet can be cold, as the hot sauce will warm it up.

HOW TO PRESSURE COOK THE MILLET IN ADVANCE

Start the pressure cooker on medium heat or use the sauté option if available. Add 1 cup (200 g) of millet and toast until fragrant. Carefully add 2 cups (475 ml) of water, cover, and pressure cook for 8 to 10 minutes. Release the pressure naturally. Take the lid off and fluff with a fork. Store in containers in the fridge for up to 3 days. This way of cooking gives millet a texture similar to couscous, and it's perfect when replacing rice or for salads. If you serve it next to a hot dish like the above, there's no need to warm it up. The hot sauce will warm up and hydrate the millet.

FIVE-SPICE BEEF RIBS WITH PARSNIP AND CELERIAC PURÉE IN A PRESSURE COOKER

The quintessential comfort dinner, this pressure cooked ribs recipe is perfect for a regular weekend dinner, but it is also a great dish to impress guests or for a holiday treat. The purée is creamy and flavorful, and the fall-off-the-bone ribs and sauce are rich and very tasty. It's easy to make, and a lot of the cooking time is actually passive time. Serve it with a mixed green salad or fermented vegetables.

Preparation time:
15 minutes

Cooking time:
1 hour

Serves:
4

FOR THE RIBS:

About 3 pounds (1.4 kg) beef short ribs (or about 2 ribs per person)

2 teaspoons five-spice blend

1 teaspoon salt

½ teaspoon freshly ground pepper

2–3 tablespoons (28 to 45 ml) extra-virgin olive oil

2 big red onions, halved and sliced

4 big garlic cloves, smashed and chopped

4 tablespoons (60 ml) coconut aminos

2 tablespoons (28 ml) aged balsamic vinegar

2½ cups (570 ml) stock or broth (vegetable or beef), warmed

2 bay leaves

FOR THE PURÉE:

1 big celeriac (celery root)

3 medium parsnips

1 teaspoon salt

2 bay leaves

2 garlic cloves, smashed

2 sprigs fresh thyme or ¼ teaspoon dried thyme

2 tablespoons (28 ml) apple cider vinegar, divided

2 tablespoons (28 ml) extra-virgin olive oil

FOR SERVING:

Freshly ground pepper

Salt

Fresh parsley

---

1. Portion the ribs and remove the excess fat (not all!) and remove the membrane on the back of the ribs, as much as you can. Soak the ribs in cold water for a few minutes, rinse them well, and then pat dry with a paper towel.

2. Coat the ribs with the five-spice blend, salt, and pepper.

3. Start the pressure cooker on medium heat or use the sauté option if available and add 2 to 3 tablespoons (28 to 45 ml) of olive oil to cover the bottom. When the oil is hot, add the ribs, but don't overcrowd the pan. Sear them in batches if necessary. Brown on all sides.

4. When all the ribs are browned, add them back to the pot and add the onions and garlic. Continue to sauté and stir for a few more minutes until the onions become fragrant and softened. Add the coconut aminos and balsamic vinegar and stir well. Add the stock or broth and bay leaves. Cover and pressure cook for 45 minutes and let the pressure release naturally for about 15 minutes.

5. While the ribs are cooking, peel the celeriac and cube it. I usually don't peel parsnips, but I always try to buy organic, and the skin is very thin. Do whatever feels good to you, depending on how the skin looks (the peel has a lot of flavor).

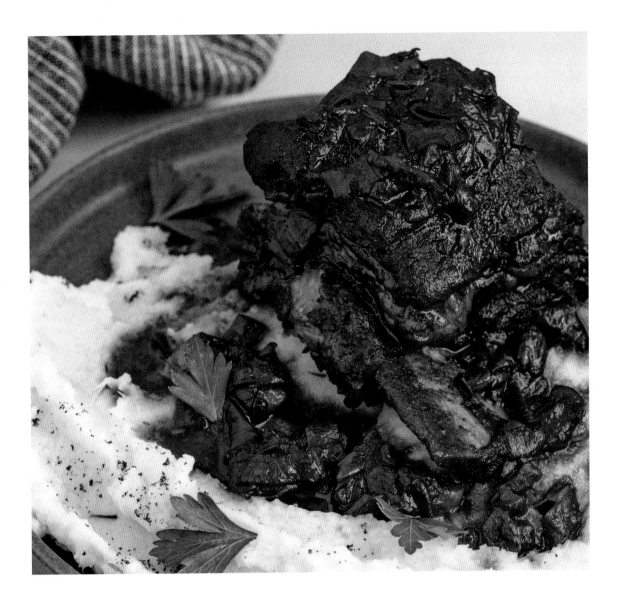

6. Rinse them in cold water and boil them with 1 teaspoon salt, bay leaves, garlic cloves, fresh (or dried) thyme, and 1 teaspoon apple cider vinegar. Simmer until fork-tender. To make the purée, drain the water (keep some just in case you need extra liquid) and discard the garlic and spices. Mash the vegetables with an immersion blender or in a blender or food processor. Add the olive oil, 1 tablespoon (15 ml) apple cider vinegar, salt, and pepper to taste.

7. To serve, plate the purée first and add the ribs and some of the sauce, sprinkle with pepper, salt if necessary, fresh parsley, and a drizzle of some of the sauce.

NOTES: The sauce will be quite fatty, but it's easy to remove some of the extra fat with a spoon. Remove the bay leaves before serving.

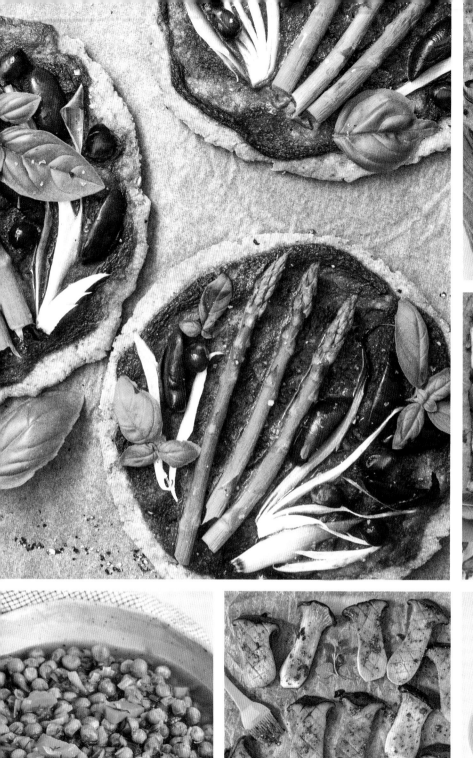
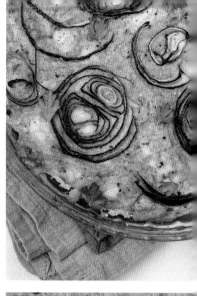
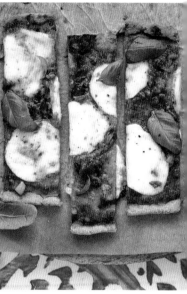
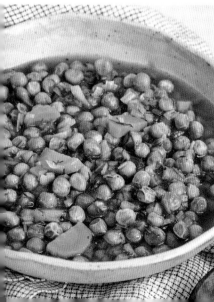
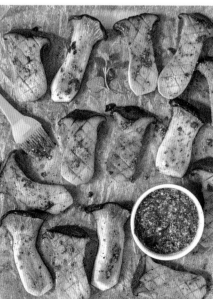
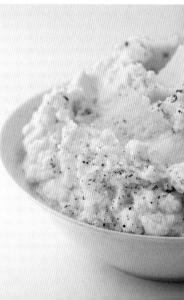

11

Vegetable Sides and Vegetarian Mains

Clockwise from top left: Asparagus Pies with Pomegranates (page 160); Curried Cauliflower and Sweet Potato Casserole (page 174); Quick Pizza Margherita Boats (from Scratch) (page 163); Cauliflower and Root Vegetable Purée with Turmeric and Chives (page 168); Oyster Mushrooms with Pesto, Millet, and Asparagus (page 152); Pressure Cooker Pea and Leek Stew (page 164)

OYSTER MUSHROOMS WITH PESTO, MILLET, AND ASPARAGUS

There are a few elements to this dish, but everything is fairly simple to prepare. I suggest you make the pesto first, whenever you have time during the day or even one day prior. You can also use any pesto you happen to have on hand. While the millet is cooking, you can prepare the mushrooms. You don't have to coordinate everything perfectly because the millet can be reheated. This is a delicious, nutritionally balanced, plant-based dinner or summer lunch.

Preparation time:
45 minutes

Cooking time:
30 minutes

Serves:
4

FOR THE PESTO:

1 bunch fresh basil leaves (cleaned and dried)

1 garlic clove, grated, or spring garlic (green garlic) if in season, finely chopped

¼–⅓ cup extra-virgin olive oil

1 ounce (30 g) toasted pine nuts

Zest of 1 organic lemon

1 or 2 tablespoons (15 to 28 ml) fresh lemon juice to taste

Salt and freshly ground pepper to taste

Optional: 2 tablespoons (10 g) grated Parmigiano Reggiano

FOR THE MILLET:

½ cup (100 g) millet

2 cups (475 ml) water

½ teaspoon salt

Pinch of nutmeg

2 tablespoons (28 g) grass-fed butter or (28 ml) extra-virgin olive oil

Freshly ground pepper

FOR THE MUSHROOMS:

1 tablespoon (4 g) fresh oregano

¼ cup (60 ml) extra-virgin olive oil

7 oyster mushrooms, clean and dried

½ teaspoon salt

Freshly ground pepper

2 tablespoons (28 ml) extra-virgin olive oil for the pan

FOR THE ASPARAGUS:

1 bunch asparagus, cleaned and woody ends trimmed

Salt and freshly ground pepper

TO MAKE THE PESTO:

This can be made in advance. Blend all the ingredients in a food processor. Store in the fridge in a glass jar with a lid for 2 to 3 days.

TO MAKE THE MILLET:

Heat a saucepan on medium heat and add the dry millet. Toast on low heat for a few minutes until it starts smelling nutty and then add the water (careful: a lot of steam will be released from the hot pan). Add the salt and a pinch of nutmeg and let simmer on low heat until all the water is absorbed. Stir occasionally. Try the millet grains, and if you feel they are not yet done, add a little bit more water and continue cooking. When ready, add some olive oil or butter, taste, and season with more salt and pepper.

TO MAKE THE MUSHROOMS:

Mix the oregano and olive oil and let it infuse for about 10 minutes. Meanwhile, slice the mushrooms in half and gently score them with a knife. Brush them with the oregano-infused olive

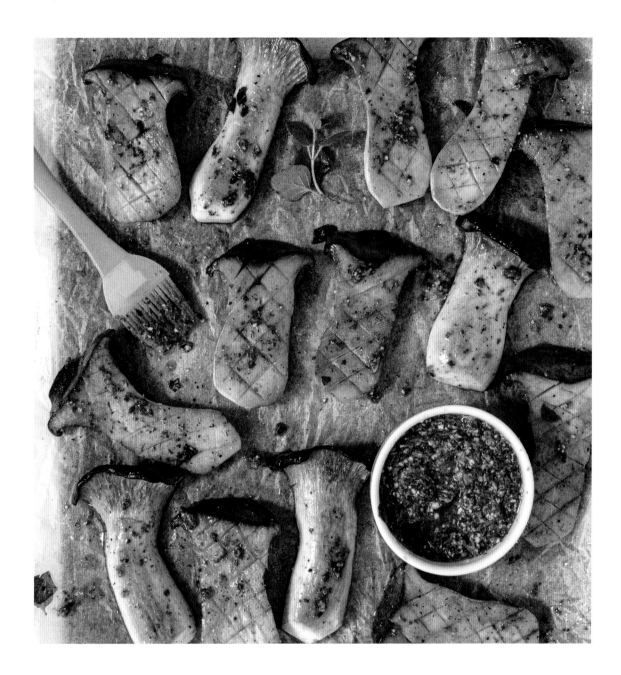

oil and season with salt and pepper. Heat some olive oil in a large skillet on medium heat and sear the mushrooms on both sides until golden brown and fragrant. Once done, place them on a platter and brush with the pesto. If you need to keep the mushrooms warm, you can keep them in the warm oven.

TO MAKE THE ASPARAGUS:
In the same pan, add the asparagus, season with salt and pepper, and sear for a few minutes, tossing a few times. They need to stay firm.

TO SERVE:
Plate the millet first, top with mushrooms and asparagus, and drizzle with pesto.

CAULIFLOWER ALFREDO PASTA

While there are plenty of cheese and dairy options we can eat if following a Plant Paradox lifestyle, creamy pasta sauces like Alfredo involve way too much dairy. So, why not take advantage of the versatility of cauliflower and make a creamy sauce that is also nutritionally dense, comforting, and healthy? Pair it with your favorite sorghum or millet lectin-free pasta.

Preparation time:
25 minutes

Cooking time:
15–20 minutes

Serves:
4

1 small head cauliflower, cut into florets, or about 5 cups (500 g) cauliflower rice

½ fennel bulb

4 big garlic cloves

2 tablespoons (25 g) French butter or 2–3 tablespoons (28 to 45 ml) extra-virgin olive oil

1 teaspoon mixed dried herbs: oregano, basil, thyme, and rosemary

¼ teaspoon ground mustard

½ teaspoon salt

¼ teaspoon freshly black pepper

Pinch of ground coriander

2 cups (475 ml) plus 3–4 tablespoons (45 to 60 ml) hemp milk, homemade (page 33) or store-bought

2 teaspoons tapioca flour

2 tablespoons (50 g) olive paste

1 teaspoon fresh lemon juice

Zest of 1 organic lemon

Optional: 2–3 tablespoons (8 to 11 g) nutritional yeast

More salt and freshly ground pepper to taste

4 portions of lectin-free pasta

Extra-virgin olive oil for serving

1. If using whole cauliflower, rice the cauliflower, fennel, and garlic in a food processor. If using cauliflower rice, finely chop the fennel and garlic.

2. Heat butter or olive oil in a large skillet and add the above mixture. Add the herbs and spices and cook on low heat for about 7 to 10 minutes or until the mix becomes soft and fragrant, making sure it is not browning or sticking to the pan.

3. Dissolve the tapioca flour in a few tablespoons (45 to 60 ml) of the hemp milk.

4. Add 2 cups (475 ml) of hemp milk to the cauliflower mix, stir well, and cook for 1 or 2 more minutes. Add the olive paste, lemon juice, lemon zest, and nutritional yeast if using and transfer everything to a blender.

5. Blend until smooth and creamy and pour back into the skillet. Add the tapioca and hemp milk mixture. Cook on low heat for about 4 minutes. Taste and add more salt, pepper, and lemon juice if necessary.

6. Prepare the lectin-free pasta according to the instructions on the package.

7. To assemble the dish, add the cooked pasta to the sauce, stir, and serve, with a drizzle of extra-virgin olive oil. You can also store this sauce in the fridge for up to 2 days for later use. Simply heat about 1 cup (235 ml) of sauce for one serving in a skillet and add one serving of cooked pasta.

CAMPING CHOPPED SALAD

Last summer we renovated our summer house in Denmark, and while working at the house, in a bit of a camping situation, I had to limit my cooking to very basic meals that didn't need much equipment and resources. But, since we were working hard, the meals had to be nutritious and satisfying. While I usually soak and pressure cook my own beans, those days I relied on canned chickpeas (canning involves pressure cooking) and ingredients that were nutritionally dense and easy to prepare such as avocado, olives, salad leaves, radishes, and fresh herbs. This is how this chopped salad was born. You can always add a boiled egg, leftover chicken, or some prosciutto on top for more protein.

Preparation time:
15 minutes

Serves:
2

4 handfuls of romaine leaves, roughly chopped

2 handfuls of bitter leaves (rucola, radicchio, or endives)

1 cup (240 g) canned chickpeas, drained and rinsed

1 avocado, chopped

4 radishes, finely sliced

1 small handful of your favorite olives

Fresh herbs, like basil or chives

3 tablespoons (45 ml) extra-virgin olive oil

Fresh lemon juice to taste

Salt and freshly ground pepper to taste

1. Add the mix of greens in a big serving bowl.

2. Top with chickpeas, avocado, radishes, olives, and fresh herbs.

3. Drizzle with olive oil and lemon juice and season with salt and pepper to taste.

MISO FONIO BOWL AND ROASTED VEGETABLES

Although new to the Western diet, fonio is an ancient small grain, a cousin of millet and native to West Africa. In addition to being a lectin-free and gluten-free grain, fonio is a powerhouse of nutrition. What is also great is that fonio needs only 3 minutes to cook. Prepare the elements of this bowl in advance and you can have a few meals or side dishes ready for the week. While it can be served cold, fonio can also be easily reheated with just a small quantity of water.

Preparation time:
20 minutes

Cooking time:
20 minutes

Serves:
4

FOR THE FONIO:

½ cup (90 g) fonio

1 tablespoon (15 ml) extra-virgin olive oil

1 cup (235 ml) water

1 teaspoon white miso paste

¼ teaspoon salt or to taste

FOR THE VEGETABLES:

20 medium Brussels sprouts

16 medium button mushrooms

2 small red onions or shallots

3 garlic cloves, whole and unpeeled

½ teaspoon dried oregano

½ teaspoon salt

¼ teaspoon freshly ground pepper

2–3 tablespoons (28 to 45 ml) extra-virgin olive oil

FOR SERVING:

4 tablespoons (60 ml) extra-virgin olive oil

2–3 tablespoons (28 to 45 ml) aged balsamic vinegar

¼ cup (20 g) ground walnuts

Sea salt flakes and freshly ground pepper for finishing

1. Preheat the oven to 400°F (200°C, or gas mark 6) and prepare a large baking sheet.

2. Clean and pat dry the vegetables. Thinly slice the Brussels sprouts and cut the mushrooms in halves or quarters, depending how big they are. Slice the onions into thin wedges.

3. Add all the vegetables onto the baking tray, season with the spices and olive oil, and toss well.

4. Roast for 15 to 20 minutes or until the vegetables soften or are cooked to your taste.

5. While the vegetables are roasting, prepare the fonio.

6. Add the fonio to a warm saucepan and add 1 tablespoon (15 ml) of olive oil. Toast for a few minutes and then add the water. Bring to a boil, let simmer for about 1 minute, and then turn the heat off. Let the fonio rest for a few minutes before you fluff it with a fork and add the miso paste and salt to your taste.

7. Remove the garlic cloves from the vegetable tray. Peel them, finely chop, and return to the vegetable mix.

8. Combine the fonio and vegetables in a big mixing bowl. Season with extra-virgin olive oil and aged balsamic vinegar and serve. Top with the ground walnuts and more balsamic vinegar if desired. Finish with sea salt flakes and pepper.

ROASTED CABBAGE WITH CRISPY CHICKPEAS AND TAHINI SAUCE

Full disclosure: I ate a similar dish in a restaurant in Denmark, and I loved it so much that I wanted to be able to make it at home. I re-created the elements of the dish from memory and the result is this. It can make a delicious side dish or a vegan main dish that is nutritious, tasty, and satisfying.

Preparation time:
15 minutes

Cooking time:
40 minutes

Serves:
2–4

FOR THE CABBAGE:

1 small to medium red cabbage

2 tablespoons (28 ml) extra-virgin olive oil

½ teaspoon salt

Freshly ground pepper

¼ teaspoon fennel seeds

¼ teaspoon dried dill

FOR THE CHICKPEAS:

1 heaping (164 g) cup pressure cooked chickpeas (drained)

4–6 spring onions or 1 red onion, finely chopped

3 garlic cloves, whole and lightly smashed

½ teaspoon salt

Freshly ground pepper

2 tablespoons (28 ml) extra-virgin olive oil

FOR THE TAHINI SAUCE:

2 tablespoons (30 g) tahini paste

½ teaspoon fresh lemon juice

¼ teaspoon local or raw honey or yacon syrup

Few teaspoons (15 ml) cold water (added one by one until you get the desired consistency)

Pinch of salt if the tahini is not already salted

FOR SERVING:

Fresh dill

Sea salt flakes and freshly ground pepper to taste

1. Preheat the oven to 400°F (200°C, or gas mark 6). You need two casserole-type baking dishes that can fit in the oven next to each other.

2. Wash and cut the cabbage into wedges. The number will depend on how big your cabbage is. A sugarloaf cabbage is pretty small, so it will make four wedges. A round cabbage will make six wedges.

3. Add the cabbage to a baking dish, drizzle with olive oil, season with salt and pepper, fennel seeds, and dried dill, and roast for 35 to 40 minutes. You can add a little water in the last 15 minutes if the pan looks too dry.

4. Add the cooked chickpeas to another baking dish that will fit next to the cabbage, add the onions and garlic, season with salt and pepper, drizzle with olive oil, toss, and put in the oven. It will need about 35 minutes to get crispy (they are not totally crispy, but pretty dry compared to the boiled ones).

5. While the veggies are cooking, make the tahini sauce. Add the tahini to a small bowl with the lemon juice and honey, start mixing, preferably with a mini hand mixer or a fork, and start adding cold water, 1 teaspoon at a time, and continue until it becomes creamy and easy to drizzle. The final consistency is up to you. If the tahini is not salted, taste and see if it needs a pinch of salt.

6. When the cabbage and chickpeas are ready, add the cabbage wedges to a serving platter, layer the chickpeas on top, drizzle on the tahini sauce, and sprinkle with fresh dill. If everything is well seasoned, you won't need extra salt, but if it needs some, use sea salt flakes.

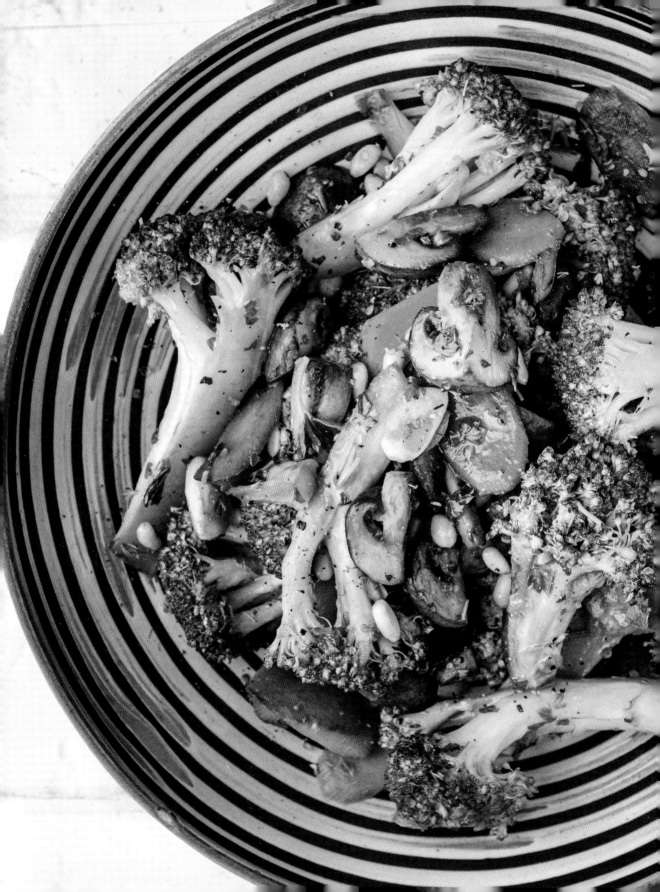

MEDITERRANEAN-STYLE STIR-FRY WITH GARLIC AND OREGANO

Sometimes, we complicate things too much and forget that the best meals are also the simplest. I ordered this dish in a Greek restaurant, and I was so impressed with the taste and how satisfying it was, I tried to re-create it at home. For some extra flavor, you can sprinkle with Parmigiano Reggiano or goat cheese. Serve it as a vegetarian main dish or as a side dish to chicken or beef.

Preparation time:
15 minutes

Cooking time:
15 minutes

Serves:
2

2 tablespoons (28 ml) extra-virgin olive oil

½ broccoli crown (about 15 small florets)

8 medium brown mushrooms, quartered (other mushrooms can also be used)

2 small carrots, sliced at an angle

3–4 garlic cloves, smashed

1 teaspoon dried oregano

½ teaspoon salt, or more to taste

½ teaspoon freshly ground pepper

1 small handful of pine nuts

1 small handful of chopped fresh parsley

Fresh lemon juice or balsamic vinegar

1. Heat a big skillet with olive oil on medium heat and add the broccoli, mushrooms, carrots, and the smashed (but whole) garlic cloves. Stir well so the veggies get coated with oil. Sauté on medium heat for about 5 minutes or until the skillet gets very dry.

2. Add a little bit of water so the veggies don't burn or stick to the bottom. Add the oregano, salt, and pepper. Let the veggies cook with the steam from the added water. It takes about 10 to 15 minutes in total or until the broccoli and carrots are done to your likeness (you can always add a few extra tablespoons [45 to 60 ml] of water).

3. In the meantime, toast the pine nuts in a separate skillet on low heat for a few minutes until they form golden brown spots and are fragrant.

4. Add the pine nuts, fresh parsley, and a squeeze of lemon juice or a drizzle of balsamic vinegar.

5. Serve as a main meal or as a side.

ASPARAGUS PIES WITH POMEGRANATES

The past few years, there was a social media trend of beautifully decorated flatbread, pizza, focaccia, or even tortillas. There is something appealing about food looking pretty. So, if you are in the mood to create something beautiful for the eyes, I invite you to make these mini pizzas. Of course, you can use any pesto you want, but I love asparagus and this combination of ingredients. You can use any of the pizza crusts or flatbreads in this book or store-bought ones. If you want to go the extra mile, add some fresh mozzarella. This recipe is also low in histamines.

Preparation time:
25 minutes

Cooking time:
10–15 minutes

Serves:
4

4 small precooked pizza crusts, flatbreads, or tortillas

12 asparagus spears, woody ends removed

1 tablespoon (15 ml) extra-virgin olive oil

1 cup Basil and Asparagus Pesto with Pistachios (page 86)

1 red onion, sliced

10 Kalamata olives, pit removed and sliced

1 generous handful of fresh basil leaves

½ cup (87 g) pomegranate arils

½ teaspoon dried oregano

Sea salt flakes

Optional: Tabasco Red Pepper Sauce

1. If the pizza crusts are frozen, thaw them in the oven at 400°F (200°C, or gas mark 6), making sure you don't overcook or burn them. If you are using fresh tortillas or flatbreads, you don't need to thaw them or warm them up in the oven.

2. Toss the asparagus with the olive oil.

3. Spread a generous layer of pesto on top of the crust and arrange the asparagus, red onion, and olives on top (see photo for inspiration).

4. Bake at 400°F (200°C, or gas mark 6) for about 8 minutes.

5. Remove from the oven and garnish with fresh basil leaves and pomegranate arils. Sprinkle with oregano and sea salt flakes and add a few drops of Tabasco Red Pepper Sauce if you want a little spice.

6. Serve immediately.

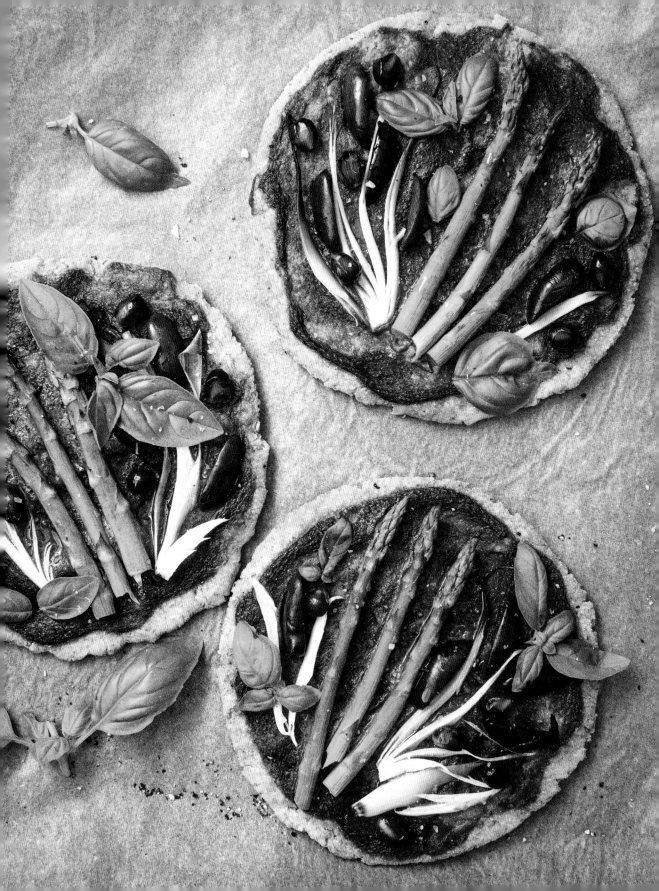

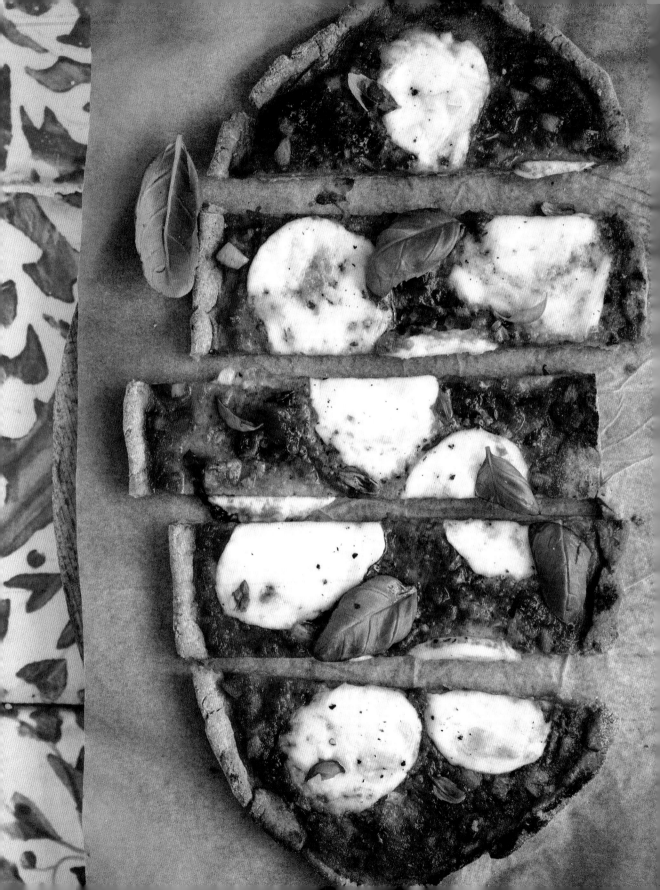

QUICK PIZZA MARGHERITA BOATS (from Scratch)

Tomatoes are not a staple in our home anymore, but every now and then, especially when we have access to local, fresh heirloom tomatoes, we like to put them to good use. My parents preserve their own tomatoes for the winter and freeze them in casseroles. They are, of course, peeled and deseeded. You will also find good quality Italian canned tomatoes, without peels and seeds. San Marzano are the best for Margherita sauce, but I use what we grow. Considering you will make the sauce and the pizza crust from scratch, these are incredibly easy and quick to make. I like to make them for Sunday brunch.

Preparation time:
30 minutes

Cooking time:
13 minutes

Serves:
4

FOR THE TOMATO SAUCE:

1 tablespoon (15 ml) extra-virgin olive oil

3 garlic cloves, minced

1 cup (180 g) peeled and deseeded tomatoes, finely chopped or minced (or use canned tomatoes, where the only ingredient is tomatoes)

½ teaspoon dried oregano

½ teaspoon salt

Freshly ground pepper

About 10 basil leaves

FOR THE PIZZA CRUSTS:

2 pizza crusts made with the Super Easy Focaccia Bread recipe (page 54)

FOR ASSEMBLING THE PIZZA:

Tomato sauce (everything that you make above)

4½ ounces (125 g) fresh buffalo mini mozzarella, cut into halves

Sea salt flakes and freshly ground pepper to taste

A few fresh basil leaves

A drizzle of extra-virgin olive oil

1. To make the tomato sauce: Heat the olive oil in a saucepan, add the garlic, cook for just 15 seconds, and then add the tomatoes. Simmer on low heat until the water evaporates, and it gets a thicker consistency. When it is almost done, add the rest of the ingredients, simmer for 1 more minute, and set aside.

2. While the tomatoes cook, make the pizza crust: Make the Super Easy Focaccia Bread recipe. Divide in two and roll out each portion into an oval shape, about 10 inches (25 cm) long and 5½ inches (13 cm) wide. Lift the edges slightly. To make it easy to transfer the dough onto the baking sheet, I add the first crust with the parchment paper I rolled it on, do the same with the next one, and just cut the excess paper. Poke holes with a fork on the entire surface and bake for about 7 to 8 minutes.

3. Remove the crusts from the oven, add the tomato sauce, arrange the mozzarella balls on top, and continue to bake for about 8 more minutes.

4. When done, remove from the oven, season with sea salt flakes, pepper, and fresh basil leaves, and drizzle with olive oil. Serve immediately.

PRESSURE COOKER PEA AND LEEK STEW

Yes, you can occasionally eat peas if you pressure cook them. When I was in college, one of my roommates was bringing home cooked food every week, and this pea stew was very often in the menu. She did share the love with us, and I was happy because I absolutely loved this dish. When I smell and taste it now, it brings me back to that time and always reminds me of her. My parents were much further away and we didn't have a kitchen, so her food was the only home-cooked food I would have. Have it as it is, next to some roasted artichoke hearts, or serve it as a side dish to chicken, pork, sausages, or any other meat. It also pairs well with a few crumbles of buffalo or goat cheese on top. I like to make a big batch because it freezes well.

Preparation time:
15 minutes

Cooking time:
15 minutes

Serves:
6–8

2 leeks, cleaned and sliced (the white and light green part)

2 carrots, sliced

3 tablespoons (45 ml) extra-virgin olive oil

2 garlic cloves, minced

½ teaspoon fennel seeds

1¾ pounds (800 g) frozen peas

½ teaspoon ground coriander

1½ teaspoons salt

¼ teaspoon freshly ground pepper

½ teaspoon paprika

1 bay leaf

1 cup (180 g) peeled and deseeded tomatoes (fresh or canned)

1 cup (235 ml) hot water

2 teaspoons tapioca flour dissolved in 2 tablespoons (28 ml) cold water

1 big bunch dill, chopped

1. Finely slice the leeks and carrot and sauté them in olive oil in your pressure cooker pot for about 7 to 10 minutes, until translucent. Don't let the leeks brown.

2. Next, add the garlic and fennel seeds, stir, and sauté for a couple more minutes.

3. Add the peas and the rest of the spices and sauté for about 5 minutes, stirring frequently.

4. Add the tomatoes, stir well, cook for a few more minutes, and add the water.

5. Cover and pressure cook for 4 minutes. Let the pressure release naturally and uncover.

6. Turn the heat on again and add the tapioca flour and water mixture, stir well, and let cook for 2 minutes.

7. Add the fresh dill and season more to taste. Remove the bay leaf before serving.

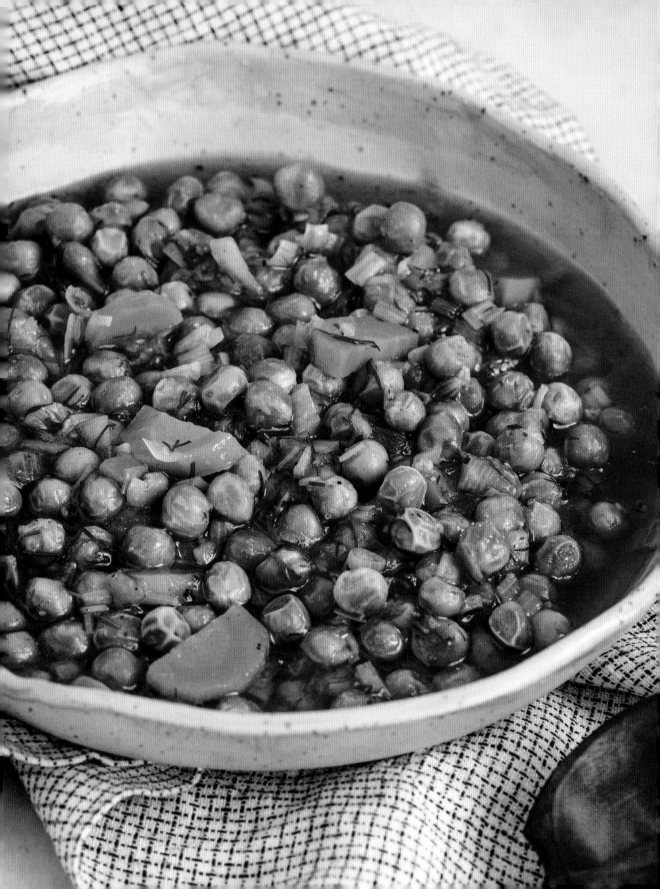

MILLET STUFFING

Classic stuffing is made with bread and has little nutritional value while being a carb and lectin bomb. Try this millet stuffing recipe instead. It makes for a nutritious side dish for your holiday feast or for any day, really. With all the vegetables and fresh herbs, this millet stuffing has similar flavors to the traditional one but is much healthier. This is also a dish that can be made in advance and stored in the refrigerator for a few days or even frozen. To warm up or thaw, rehydrate with a little bit of water or stock and warm in the oven. The millet is made quick and easy in a pressure cooker.

Preparation time:
30 minutes

Cooking time:
50 minutes

Serves:
6

FOR THE MILLET:
1 cup (200 g) millet
2 cups (475 ml) water
¼ teaspoon sea salt

FOR THE STUFFING:
1 leek, well cleaned and chopped
1 big yellow onion, chopped
3 big celery ribs, sliced
1 fennel bulb with stalks, roughly chopped
5 tablespoons (75 ml) extra-virgin olive oil
½ teaspoon sea salt
¼ teaspoon freshly ground pepper
1 tablespoon (3 g) chopped fresh sage
1 tablespoon (2 g) chopped fresh thyme
1 tablespoon (2 g) chopped fresh rosemary
2 pastured eggs
3 tablespoons (45 ml) filtered water
1 tablespoon (15 ml) extra-virgin olive oil
More salt and freshly ground pepper to taste

1. Rinse the millet in cold water and place the millet in a pressure cooker. Add 2 cups (475 ml) of water and ¼ teaspoon sea salt, seal the pot, and cook on high pressure for 11 minutes. When the program is done, release the pressure manually, take the lid off, and fluff with a fork.

2. Preheat the oven to 350°F (180°C, or gas mark 4).

3. Sauté all the vegetables in olive oil until soft and fragrant. Add the fresh herbs and spices, combine well, sauté for a few more minutes, and take off the heat.

4. Beat the eggs with 3 tablespoons (45 ml) of water.

5. Combine the cooked millet with the sautéed vegetables and herbs and add the eggs.

6. Pour the mixture into a baking or casserole dish and bake for 35 minutes.

7. After 20 minutes, remove from the oven and toss the mixture again, trying to mix the parts at the bottom (where most of the egg is) with parts at the top. Put back in and bake until the time is done.

8. Remove from the oven, generously drizzle with olive oil, add salt and pepper to taste, and serve warm.

9. This meal can also be reheated. To make in advance, freeze and rewarm in the oven, rehydrating with a little bit of vegetable or chicken stock.

CREAMY LENTIL AND VEGETABLE STEW

Pressure cooking lentils kills most of the nasty lectins and makes this nutritious staple easier on your digestive system. The only problem when pressure cooking lentils is that they easily lose shape and get mushy. A solution is to use French green lentils, as they hold their shape well. I also like to pressure cook lentils as part of my meal prep and have them ready to add to this meal.

Preparation time:
20 minutes

Cooking time:
30 minutes

Serves:
4

4 tablespoons (60 ml) extra-virgin olive oil (for sautéing)

1 medium yellow or sweet onion, chopped

1 leek, cleaned and chopped

8 small button mushrooms, quartered

1 medium parsnip, peeled and cut into small cubes

1 medium kohlrabi, peeled and cut into small cubes

1 small celeriac (celery root), peeled and cut into small cubes

5 garlic cloves, smashed and minced

1½ teaspoons salt (start with 1 teaspoon and add more if necessary to your taste)

½ tablespoon herbs de Provence

¼ teaspoon freshly ground black pepper, or more to taste

1 baby bok choy, chopped

2 cups (396 g) pressure cooked lentils (page 18 or used canned lentils)

2 cups (475 ml) hot water

3 tablespoons (45 ml) extra-virgin olive oil (for the blending)

1 handful of fresh parsley

1 squeeze of fresh lemon

1. Have a pot full of hot water on the stove.

2. Add the olive oil to a big stew pot and add chopped onion, leek, mushrooms, parsnip, kohlrabi, and celeriac. Stir well and sauté for 10 minutes on low heat, stirring occasionally so it doesn't stick. If it gets too dry and starts sticking too much to the pan, add 2 to 3 tablespoons (28 to 45 ml) of hot water.

3. After 10 minutes, when all the veggies soften up and get fragrant, add the garlic, salt, herbs de Provence, and pepper. Stir well and cook for 5 more minutes.

4. Add the boy choy and a few tablespoons (45 to 60 ml) of water and stir and cook for a few minutes.

5. Add the lentils and 2 cups (475 ml) of water and cook for about 5 more minutes, stirring occasionally. Turn the heat off.

6. Remove about ½ of the lentil mixture, or at least ⅓, and blend with 3 tablespoons (45 ml) of olive oil. Add back into the stew pot, stir everything together, and turn the heat on and simmer for a couple more minutes. Add the fresh parsley. Adjust for salt and pepper, add a squeeze of lemon juice, and serve.

CAULIFLOWER AND ROOT VEGETABLE PURÉE WITH TURMERIC AND CHIVES

A purée or mash is always the perfect side dish. I got all my family converted to this one, and we often make it to replace the white potato purée. This pressure-cooked recipe goes with everything meat or fish, but you can serve it with sautéed asparagus or mushrooms and a green salad for a complete plant-based meal.

Preparation time:
15 minutes

Cooking time:
10 minutes

Serves:
4

½ big cauliflower head (or 1 small one)

1 big parsnip, peeled

1 small celeriac (celery root), peeled

1 medium sweet potato, peeled

2 tablespoons (28 ml) extra-virgin olive oil

4–5 garlic cloves, smashed

½ teaspoon mustard seeds

4–5 allspice berries (or use ¼ teaspoon ground allspice)

1 teaspoon ground turmeric

1 cup (235 ml) water

1 tablespoon (15 ml) apple cider vinegar

½ teaspoon salt

¼ teaspoon freshly ground pepper

1–2 tablespoons (15 to 28 ml) extra-virgin olive oil

More salt and freshly ground pepper for finishing

½ teaspoon dried chives or a small handful of fresh

1. Prepare all the vegetables and cut them into cubes. Leave the cauliflower in big florets (bigger than the chunks of root vegetables).

2. Add the olive oil to a pressure cooker on low-to-medium heat or use the sauté option if available and add the garlic, mustard seeds, and allspice. Sauté for 2 to 3 minutes.

3. Add the turmeric and all the veggies. Stir well so all the veggies get coated with the spices and oil and add the water, apple cider vinegar, salt, and pepper.

4. Cover and pressure cook for 3 minutes.

5. When the time is done, let the pressure release naturally for about 5 to 10 minutes. Release the rest manually if there is more.

6. Remove more than half of the liquid and blend everything with an immersion blender or transfer to a normal blender.

7. Add some olive oil, taste for salt and pepper, blend again or mix well, and add the chives.

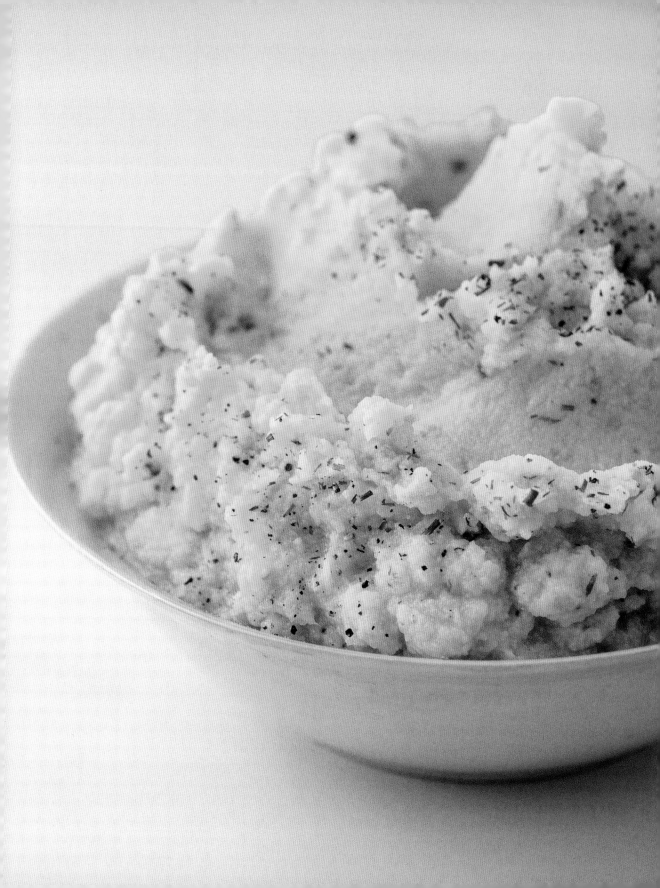

AYURVEDA-INSPIRED LECTIN-LIGHT KITCHARI

This is the perfect meal when you feel like your digestive system is easily bothered and needs a break. Kitchari, which is a mixture of two grains, usually mung beans or lentils and rice, is a soothing Ayurvedic food. While the traditional way of preparation can be hard on people with lectin sensitivity, there is a way to make this dish lectin-light by pressure cooking the lentils and rice. The texture of this meal will be porridge-like, so all the ingredients have to be cooked very well. This, in combination with the specific mix of spices, will make this meal soothing and healing. A kitchari cleanse means you are eating the same food, for every meal, for three days. I combine it with intermittent fasting and eat two kitchari meals every day for three days.

While eating leftovers is not recommended in Ayurveda, you can eat this kitchari the next day or at the next meal if cooking for every meal doesn't fit your lifestyle. This a plant-based, lectin-light, nourishing, and satisfying meal.

Preparation time:
40 minutes

Cooking time:
40 minutes

Serves:
2

½ cup (84 g) black rice or (93 g) Indian basmati rice (preferably organic)

1 cup (192 g) red lentils

A few cups (weight will vary) of seasonal, easy-to-digest vegetables such as cauliflower, celery, purslane, zucchini (no peel and seeds), fennel bulb, asparagus, sweet potato, broccoli, or spinach

1 tablespoon (14 g) coconut oil (extra-virgin olive oil or ghee can be used)

1. Rinse the rice and pressure cook it for 10 minutes, with enough water. Allow a natural release of pressure. Drain excess water and let it cool. Rice is better digested and provides the resistant starch benefits if it's cooled before eating or reheating.

2. Rinse the lentils and pressure cook for 4 minutes, with enough water. Allow a natural release of pressure. Scoop the lentils out and discard the liquid. They will get pretty mushy, but that's perfect for this dish. You can do this in advance to allow the rice time to cool before reheating.

3. Chop the cauliflower into small pieces. Chop the rest of the veggies. Whatever veggies you are using, it's important they are well cooked, so add them in the order of the time they need to cook. Cauliflower would take longer than zucchini and asparagus for example. The leafy greens can be added in the last 10 minutes.

Spices: 1 teaspoon ground cumin, ½ teaspoon ground coriander, 1 teaspoon mustard seeds, 1 teaspoon fennel seeds, 1 teaspoon grated ginger, ½ teaspoon ground turmeric, and ½ teaspoon fenugreek powder

2½–3 (570 to 700 ml) cups water

Fresh cilantro for serving

4. Heat the coconut oil on medium heat, add the cumin, coriander, mustard seeds, and fennel seeds, and cook for a few minutes until the oil gets fragrant (do not burn the spices as they get bitter).

5. Add the cauliflower and other hard veggies (celery, carrots, or fennel), stir well, and add the ginger, turmeric, and fenugreek.

6. Add 2½ cups (570 ml) of hot water over the veggies, or enough to cover them, and simmer for about 20 minutes or until cauliflower is tender.

7. Add the rice and the lentils. If you use any tender green leaves like spinach, you can add them now. Add salt to taste. Simmer for about 10 more minutes. Add more water if necessary. The consistency should be creamy and porridge-like. Keep in mind that when it cools down, the ingredients absorb more liquid.

8. Serve with fresh cilantro. Add more salt if necessary.

CREAMY SORGHUM RISOTTO WITH MUSHROOMS AND ARUGULA

Sorghum is an excellent replacement for rice when making risotto. The best way to make this meal quick and easy is to use precooked sorghum. I prefer to cook it in the pressure cooker since it's much faster than stovetop cooking. It takes only 12 minutes and can easily be stored in the refrigerator for a few days and even frozen.

Preparation time:
30 minutes

Cooking time:
30 minutes

Serves:
4

2 cups (350 g) cooked sorghum

3 tablespoons (45 ml) extra-virgin olive oil

1 yellow onion, chopped

2 cups (108 g) mushrooms, chanterelle or any mix of mushrooms you have, chopped or sliced

2 garlic cloves, minced

1 cup (235 ml) vegetable (or chicken) stock

2 handfuls of arugula or spinach

Salt and pepper to taste (depends on how salty your stock is)

Pinch of nutmeg

¼ cup (31 g) toasted pistachios, chopped

Optional: 2–3 tablespoons (10 to 15 g) grated Parmigiano Reggiano

1. Make sure you have cooked sorghum; see page 19 for instructions on how to cook it. If you have raw pistachios, you can toast them in a skillet or in the oven, at 300°F (150°C, or gas mark 2), for about 8 minutes.

2. Heat the olive oil in a skillet or a wide-bottom pot and add the onions. Sauté on medium heat until translucent.

3. Add the mushrooms and garlic and sauté for about 5 to 8 minutes until the mushrooms become fragrant and most of the liquid evaporates.

4. Add the cooked sorghum, toss well, and start adding about ¼ cup (60 ml) of stock at a time. Turn the heat to low. When the liquid evaporates, add more stock until you finished the 1 cup (235 ml). It will take about 10 to 15 minutes.

5. Once you've used all the stock, add the arugula or spinach. Add salt and pepper to taste and a pinch of nutmeg.

6. Serve with the chopped pistachios and grated Parmigiano Reggiano if you eat dairy.

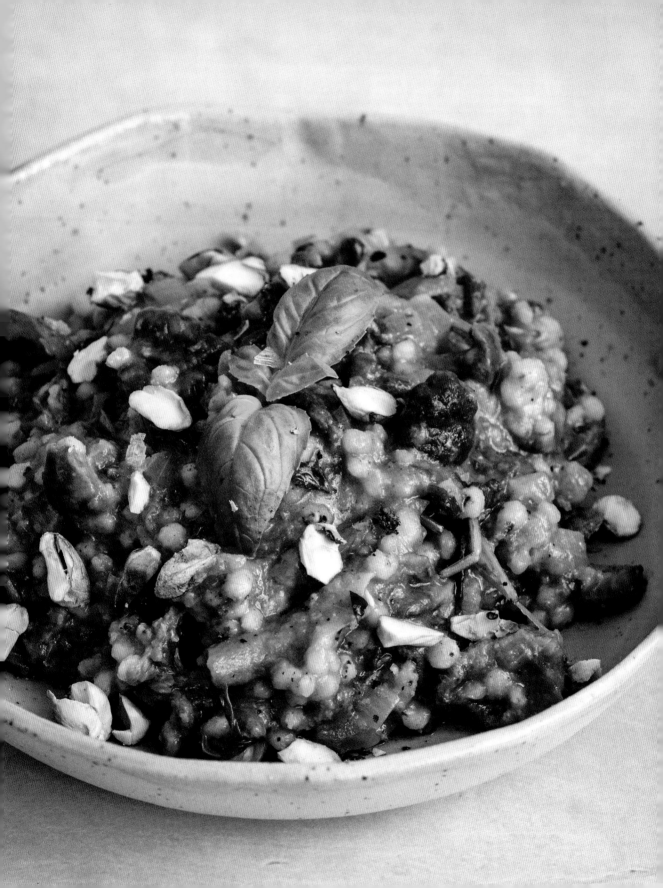

CURRIED CAULIFLOWER AND SWEET POTATO CASSEROLE

This casserole, my take on Yotam Ottolenghi's cauliflower cake, is such a versatile dish. It can make a great family breakfast, a perfect side dish, or a main meal if you are vegetarian. It goes well with fermented vegetables, like sauerkraut, or a big mixed greens salad. It can be served warm or cold and can easily be warmed in the oven. While cheese can be added if you want to, I prefer to keep this one dairy-free.

Preparation time:
25 minutes

Cooking time:
30 minutes

Serves:
6

1 head cauliflower, cut into small florets

2 small sweet potatoes

4 pastured eggs

½ cup (120 g) coconut cream

3 tablespoons (45 ml) extra-virgin olive oil

1 heaping teaspoon curry powder

1½ teaspoons salt

¼ teaspoon freshly ground pepper

1 garlic clove, grated

4–5 tablespoons (35 to 45 g) cassava flour

1 red onion, finely sliced into rings

FOR SERVING:

Fresh parsley

Freshly ground pepper

Big green salad or sauerkraut

1. Preheat the oven to 400°F (200°C, or gas mark 6) and prepare a round pie dish or any casserole-type dish. Lightly coat it with olive oil.

2. Boil or steam the cauliflower until it slightly softens but is still al dente (if you boil it, add salt to the water). Take it out, let it strain in a colander for a few minutes, and then place it onto a large platter lined with paper towels, so you get as much of the moisture out as possible.

3. While the cauliflower is cooking, peel and grate the potatoes and prepare the rest of the ingredients.

4. Combine the eggs, coconut cream, olive oil, and spices in a bowl and then add the sweet potatoes and cassava flour. Mix well.

5. Arrange the cauliflower florets in the pie dish and then pour the egg and sweet potato mixture on top.

6. Finely slice the onion into rings and place them on top (this is mostly for decoration, but the caramelized onion will add some flavor too).

7. Bake for 30 to 35 minutes until no longer soft to the touch and golden brown and let it set for about 10 minutes.

8. Garnish with fresh parsley and pepper and serve with a big green salad or sauerkraut.

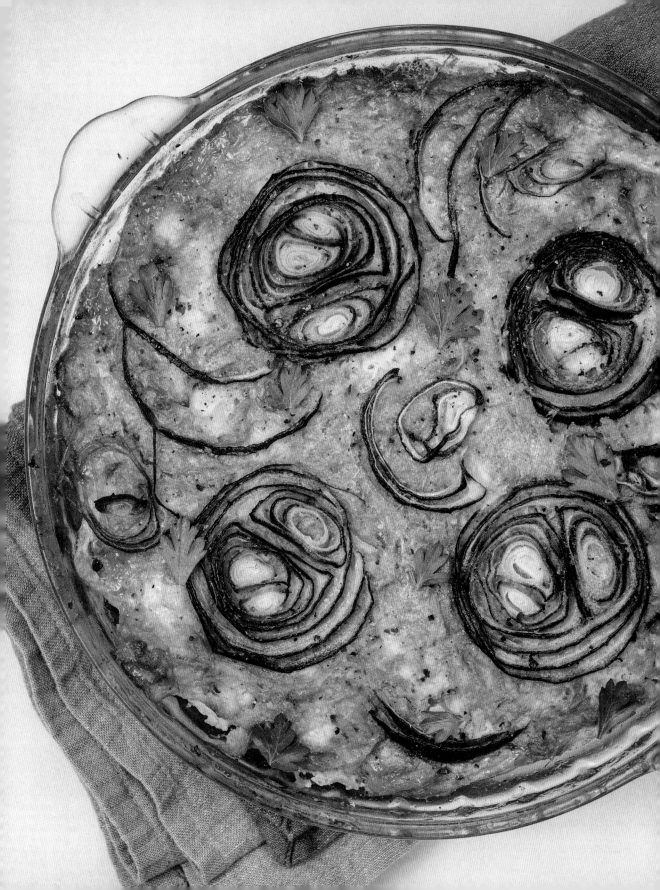

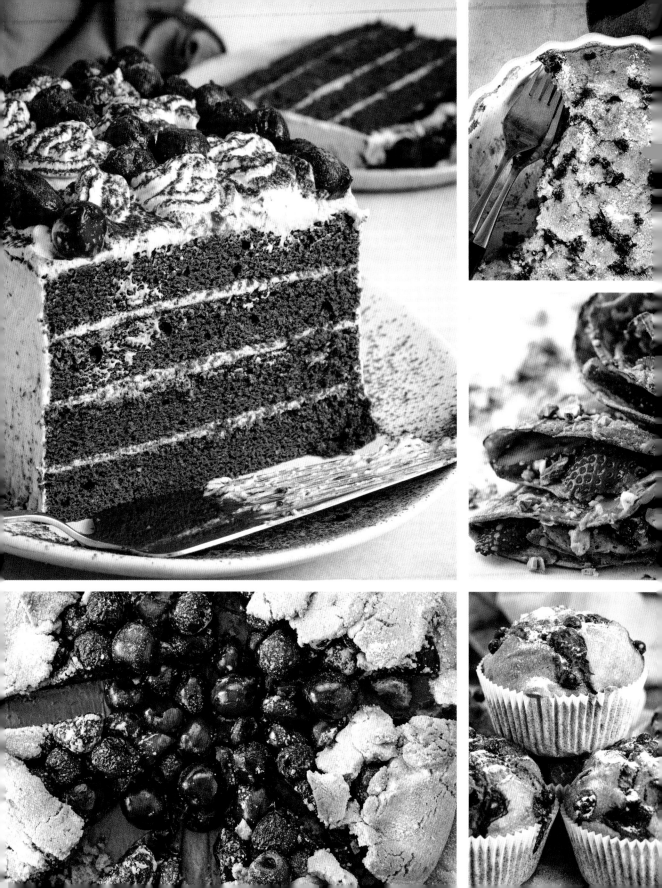

12

Sweets and Treats

Clockwise from top left: Red Velvet Cake with Mascarpone and Coconut Cream (page 186); Blackberry Clafoutis (page 181); Chestnut Crepes with Strawberries and Pistachios (page 194); Orange Gingerbread Muffins with Green Banana (page 184); Rustic Cherry Galette (page 178)

RUSTIC CHERRY GALETTE

The cherry season is the best season. After eating fresh cherries, a lectin-free and sugar-free rustic cherry galette is the next best thing. Unpretentious and easy to make, this galette is a healthy early-summer treat to share with family and friends. This galette is made with sweet cherries, but tart cherries can also be used. Just add some extra sweetener. Cherries, especially tart cherries, are rich in melatonin, a mitochondrial must-have.

Preparation time:
35 minutes

Cooking time:
35 minutes

Serves:
8

FOR THE CRUST:

1 cup (140 g) cassava flour

3 tablespoons (27 g) arrowroot or (24 g) tapioca flour

½ cup (56 g) chestnut flour

½ cup (52 g) almond flour

1 tablespoon (12 g) monk fruit sweetener or (15 g) inulin powder

¼ teaspoon salt

Zest of 1 organic lemon

2 pastured eggs

1 teaspoon pure vanilla extract

½ cup (112 g) coconut oil, softened but not melted

4 tablespoons (60 ml) ice-cold water

FOR THE FILLING:

4–5 cups (620 to 775 g) fresh cherries, pitted

2 teaspoons tapioca flour

1 tablespoon (12 g) monk fruit sweetener or (15 g) inulin powder (more if you use tart cherries)

1 tablespoon (15 ml) fresh lemon juice

Zest of 1 organic lemon

1. Preheat the oven to 350°F (180°C, or gas mark 4).

2. Combine the flours, sweetener, and salt in a food processor.

3. Add the lemon zest, eggs, vanilla, coconut oil, and water and process on high until everything gets mixed together. At this point, it will look more like a crumble.

4. Place the dough into a bowl or onto a sheet of parchment paper and start working it with your hands. It will be a hard dough at first, but it will eventually stick together. Shape the dough in a ball and let it rest in the fridge while you are preparing the filling.

5. Prepare the cherries: pit them and mix them in a bowl with the tapioca flour, sweetener, lemon juice, and lemon zest.

6. Prepare a work surface with two parchment papers and a rolling pin. Take the dough out of the fridge (it needs about 30 minutes in the fridge), knead it a little bit so it warms up, and start to flatten it on the bottom parchment paper, spreading it into a round or an oval shape. Add the parchment sheet on top and start rolling with a pin until you get a sheet about ⅛ inch (3 mm) thick. The dough might crumble a little bit on the edges, but it's easy to stick back together using your fingers. Peel the top parchment paper off and transfer the bottom one with the dough onto a baking sheet.

7. Arrange the cherry filling on top of the dough, leaving about a 1½-inch (3.8 cm) space all around on the sides. Leave some cherries out to add on top after you fold the edges.

TIP: You can make this rustic galette using other seasonal fruits.

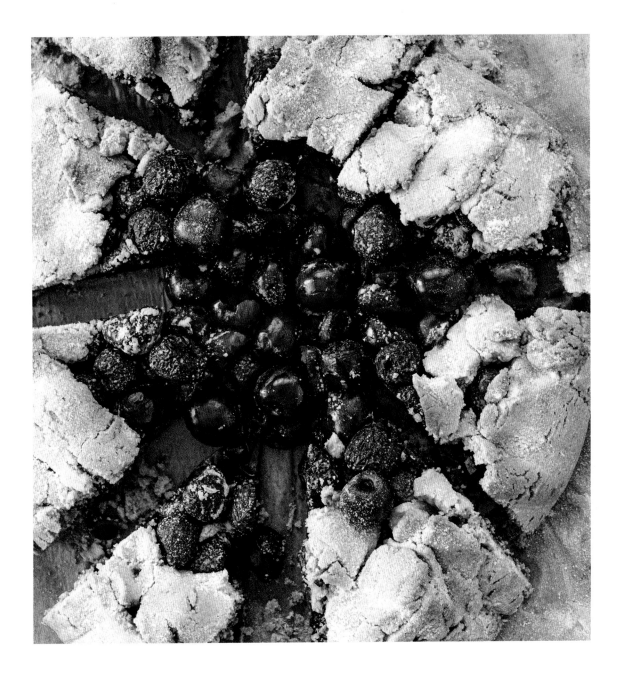

8. Fold the edges on top of the cherry filling, using the parchment paper to lift it and fold it over. Don't worry if it breaks, just stick it back together. Add the rest of the cherries in the middle.

9. Bake for about 35 minutes or until the dough and top are golden brown but keep an eye on it so it doesn't burn.

10. After taking it out of the oven, dust it with inulin powder or another powdered sweetener. Allow it to cool down slightly. Eat warm or store in the fridge for 2 to 3 days. I love it both warm and cold, but my favorite way to eat it is the second day, cold from the fridge.

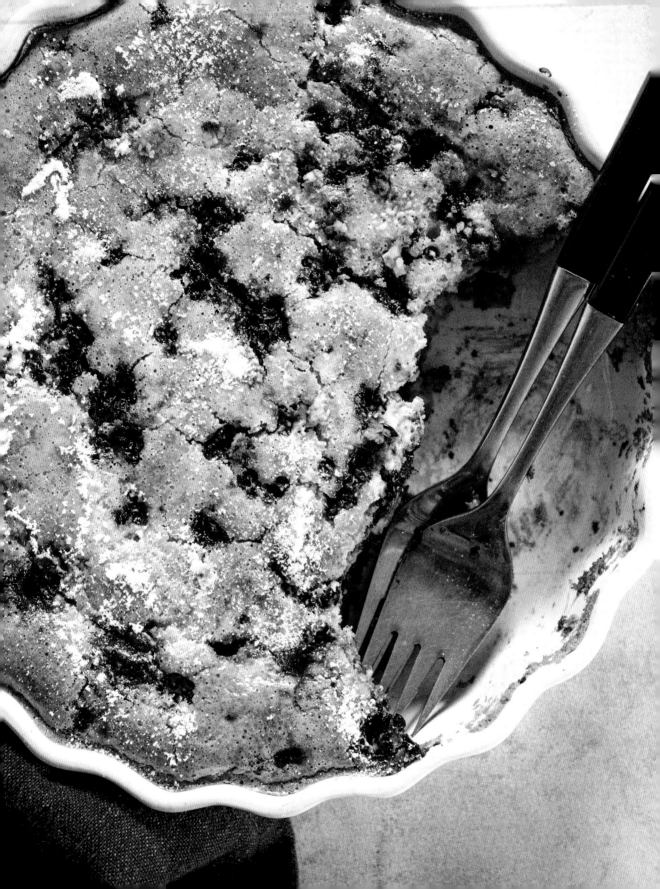

BLACKBERRY CLAFOUTIS

Wild blackberries are everywhere around our summer house in Denmark. I love picking them and putting them to good use. While clafoutis is normally made with cherries, and you can certainly use this recipe to make a cherry clafoutis, blackberries work beautifully. Use them when they are in season and it's even better if you can pick them yourself.

Preparation time:
10 minutes

Cooking time:
40 minutes

Serves:
4

1 teaspoon coconut oil for coating the baking dish

3 pastured eggs

1 cup (240 g) coconut cream

3 tablespoons (45 g) inulin powder (or another compliant sweetener), more if you have a sweet tooth

Pinch of salt

1 teaspoon pure vanilla extract

Optional: 1 teaspoon almond extract (if you like the extra almond flavor)

½ cup (52 g) almond flour (packed)

About 2–3 cups (290 to 435 g) blackberries (the more, the better)

1. Preheat the oven to 350°F (180°C, or gas mark 4) and prepare a baking dish of about 7 inches (18 cm) in diameter or something equivalent in any shape, such as a glass or metal pie dish or even a cast-iron pan. The baking dish should be coated with coconut oil.

2. Add the eggs, coconut cream, sweetener, salt, vanilla, and almond extract if using to a mixing bowl and whisk until creamy.

3. Add the almond flour and combine until all is incorporated. You should get a thick, fluffy, and creamy batter.

4. Pour the batter into the oiled baking dish, level, and place the blackberries on top, slightly pushing them down into the batter. They just need a little space in between.

5. Bake for 40 minutes until the clafoutis has set and is golden brown. You can eat it warm or cold.

APPLE GALETTE WITH HAZELNUT CRUMBLE

This apple galette is a favorite in our home during apple season. It's easy to make and delicious. While it can be eaten warm, straight from the oven, I love to eat it cold, the next day. If you want to be extra, go ahead and pair a warm slice of this galette with a compliant vanilla ice cream and dust it with a little bit of cinnamon. It will make your day.

Preparation time:
30 minutes

Cooking time:
35 minutes

Serves:
12

FOR THE CRUST:

1 cup (140 g) cassava flour

3 tablespoons (27 g) arrowroot or (24 g) tapioca flour

½ cup (56 g) chestnut flour

½ cup (52 g) almond flour

1 tablespoon (12 g) monk fruit sweetener or (15 g) inulin powder

¼ teaspoon salt

Zest of 1 organic lemon

2 pastured eggs

1 teaspoon pure vanilla extract

½ cup (112 g) coconut oil, softened but not melted

4 tablespoons (60 ml) ice-cold water

1. Preheat the oven to 350°F (180°C, or gas mark 4).

2. Combine the flours, sweetener, and salt in a food processor.

3. Add the lemon zest, eggs, vanilla, coconut oil, and water and process on high until everything gets mixed together. At this point, it will look more like a crumble.

4. Place the dough into a bowl or onto a sheet of parchment paper and start working it with your hands. It will be a hard dough at first, but it will stick together. Shape the dough in a ball and let it rest in the fridge while you are preparing the apples.

5. Prepare the apples. Cut them in half, core them, and then slice each half really thin without pulling the slices apart. Leave them cut-side down until the dough is ready (so they don't oxidize).

6. Prepare a work surface with two parchment papers and a rolling pin. Take the dough out of the fridge, knead it a little bit so it warms up, and start to flatten it on the bottom parchment paper, spreading it into a round or a rectangle. Add the parchment sheet on top and start rolling with a pin until you get a sheet about ⅛ inch (3 mm) thick. The dough might crumble a little bit on the edges, but it's easy to stick back together using your fingers. Peel the top parchment paper off and slide the bottom one with the dough onto a baking sheet.

FOR THE FILLING:

4–5 apples, depending on size (I use Gala or Fuji)

1 teaspoon cinnamon

1 tablespoon (12 g) monk fruit sweetener or (15 g) inulin powder

¼ cup (28 g) roughly ground hazelnuts or pecans

1 tablespoon (14 g) coconut oil

½ tablespoon yacon syrup

7. Arrange the apple slices on top of the dough, overlapping the slices (you take each half at a time, press down slowly, and spread it with your hand). Repeat until you fill the dough layer, leaving about a 1½-inch (3.8 cm) space all around on the sides.

8. Sprinkle the cinnamon and the sweetener on top of the apples.

9. Fold the edges on top of the apple filling, using the parchment paper to lift it and fold it over the apples. Don't worry if it breaks; just stick it back together.

10. Mix the ground hazelnuts with coconut oil and sprinkle on top of the apple center.

11. Bake for about 35 minutes or until the dough and the top are golden brown but keep an eye on it so it doesn't burn.

12. You can spread more coconut oil on the edges of the dough when it's out of the oven. Drizzle the yacon syrup over the top of the galette.

13. Let cool down slightly and eat warm or store in the fridge for up to 3 days. I love it both warm and cold, but my favorite way to eat it is the second day, cold from the fridge.

ORANGE GINGERBREAD MUFFINS WITH GREEN BANANA

These orange gingerbread muffins made with teff and tigernut flour are the perfect cold-weather treat. They smell and taste like the holidays and are soft and light and very easy to make. If you need a warm, comforting, and grounding treat that is also lectin-free, gluten-free, and sugar-free, you have to try these muffins. You won't be disappointed.

Preparation time:
25 minutes

Cooking time:
30–35 minutes

Makes:
12 muffins

WET INGREDIENTS:

4 green bananas

4 large pastured eggs (if they are small, add 1 extra)

1 cup (235 ml) extra-virgin olive oil

4 tablespoons (60 g) inulin powder (or another compliant sweetener), plus more for dusting

2 teaspoons pure vanilla extract (or ½ teaspoon vanilla powder)

½ teaspoon licorice root powder

Zest of 3 organic oranges

Pinch of salt

Spice mix: 2 teaspoons cinnamon, ½ teaspoon ground allspice, ¾ teaspoon ground cloves, ½ teaspoon ground ginger, and ¼ teaspoon nutmeg

DRY INGREDIENTS:

1 cup (140 g) teff flour

½ cup (60 g) tigernut flour

6 tablespoons (48 g) tapioca flour

2 teaspoons baking powder

ADD-ONS:

½ cup (55 g) chopped pecans, plus more for topping

1. Preheat the oven to 350°F (180°C, or gas mark 4) and line a muffin pan with muffin paper liners.

2. Blend the wet ingredients and the spices in a blender until smooth and creamy.

3. Combine the dry ingredients in a big mixing bowl.

4. Add the wet ingredients to the dry ingredients bowl and combine with a spatula, without overmixing.

5. Add the chopped pecans and fold them into the batter.

6. Fill all 12 muffin cups with batter. Top with the rest of the pecan nuts.

7. Bake for 30 to 35 minutes. They will be golden brown and no longer soft to the touch. If you are not sure if they are done, do the toothpick test: a toothpick inserted in a muffin should come out clean.

8. Remove the muffins from the oven and let them cool down for about 10 minutes before taking them out of the pan.

9. When ready, arrange them on a serving platter and dust them with inulin powder.

10. Serve them the same day or freeze them.

STRAWBERRY MILLET FLAKE COOKIES

If you miss oatmeal cookies, these can be your treat. And while there is millet in the composition, all the rest of the ingredients are keto friendly, which makes these cookies quite low in carbohydrates. The strawberries give them a little extra moisture, and we all know how well chocolate and strawberries go together. I brought these cookies to a dinner party, and everyone devoured them.

Preparation time:
15 minutes

Cooking time:
12–15 minutes

Serves:
8–10

2 pastured eggs, room temperature

⅓ cup (85 g) coconut butter, melted but not warm

⅓ cup (75 g) coconut oil, melted but not warm

⅓ cup (85 g) nut butter (I used hazelnut butter)

1½ cups (156 g) almond flour

½ cup (60 g) tigernut flour

⅔ cup (77 g) millet flakes

1 teaspoon baking powder

1 teaspoon cinnamon

¼ teaspoon nutmeg

Pinch of salt

1 teaspoon pure vanilla extract

1 tablespoon (15 g) inulin powder or other compliant sweeteners, or more to your preference

2½ ounces (70 g) dark chocolate, chopped, or chocolate chips, minimum 75% cacao (add more if your heart desires)

1 cup (170 g) chopped strawberries

1. Preheat the oven to 350°F (180°C, or gas mark 4) and take the eggs out of the fridge. Prepare a baking sheet with parchment paper.

2. Warm the oils and butter by inserting the jars into hot water or melt them any other way that is convenient for you, mix them well, and let cool. Make sure they won't be too warm when you mix them with the eggs. (Coconut butter tends to be very hard. That's why it needs to be melted first so you can measure it and combine it with the rest of the oils and nut butter.)

3. Combine all the flours, millet flakes, baking powder, cinnamon, nutmeg, and salt in a bowl.

4. In a bigger bowl, combine the melted butters together and add the eggs, vanilla, and sweetener and whisk.

5. Add the dry mixture to the wet and mix the dough with your hands. The dough might look a little crumbly, but once you shape it in your warm hands, it'll stick together.

6. Add most of the chocolate to the dough, combine, and leave some chocolate to add on top. Fold in the strawberries.

7. Shape the dough into about 15 balls. Place them on the baking sheet and gently press them down, without making them too thin. Gently stick the sides back together if they split too much.

8. Bake for about 12 minutes if you make them without the strawberries and about 20 minutes if you make them with the strawberries (they need more time due to the extra moisture). Remove from the oven and allow them to cool down. You can store them in an airtight container on the counter if it's not too hot in the kitchen or in a cool place. Keep in the fridge for up to 3 days or better yet, freeze them. These cookies freeze and thaw very well, and I actually prefer the texture after they've been frozen.

RED VELVET CAKE WITH MASCARPONE AND COCONUT CREAM

This is the easiest birthday cake you will ever make. The layers are all made at once in a shallow sheet pan. Since the layers are thin, look for a half-pan measuring about 10 x 13 inches (25 x 35 cm). If you want to make a bigger cake, double the quantity and use two sheet pans or one that's double the size. Don't worry if the color of the cake is not exactly red. The original red velvet cake had the same color, given by the chemical reaction between cacao and apple cider vinegar (or buttermilk). And, if you still want a little bit of red color, use 1 or 2 teaspoons of beetroot powder. This is a moist, fluffy cake that tastes like some of the best red velvet cakes I've had.

Preparation time:
35 minutes

Cooking time:
15 minutes

Serves:
6

WET INGREDIENTS:

1 cup (240 g) coconut cream or (235 ml) full-fat coconut milk

2 tablespoons (28 ml) apple cider vinegar

3 pastured eggs

⅓ cup (80 ml) extra-virgin olive oil

4 tablespoons (60 g) inulin powder (or another compliant sweetener)

1 cup (235 ml) warm water

DRY INGREDIENTS:

1 cup (112 g) chestnut flour

¾ cup (78 g) almond flour

⅓ cup (40 g) tigernut flour

2 tablespoons (16 g) tapioca flour

¼ teaspoon salt

2 tablespoons (10 g) cacao powder

3 tablespoons (24 g) carob powder

2 teaspoons pure vanilla extract

2 teaspoons baking soda

Optional: 1–2 teaspoons beetroot powder, for a more intense red color

FOR THE MASCARPONE AND COCONUT CREAM:

2 cups (250 g) mascarpone cream (cold)

5 tablespoons (75 g) coconut cream (cold)

2 tablespoons (30 g) inulin powder (or another compliant powdered sweetener)

1 teaspoon pure vanilla extract

FOR DECORATION:

Carob, cacao, and/or aronia berry (chokeberry) or beetroot powder

---

1. Mix the coconut cream or milk with the apple cider vinegar. Let them sit for 15 minutes while you are preparing the rest of the ingredients.

2. Preheat the oven to 350°F (180°C, or gas mark 4) and line a sheet pan (shallow baking tray) with parchment paper (see above dimensions).

3. Mix all the dry ingredients in a big bowl. You can sift the entire mix if you don't want any clumps. The chestnut flour, cacao, and carob are the most likely to form clumps.

4. Whisk all the wet ingredients in another bowl, including the coconut cream mix, until well combined.

5. Add the wet ingredients over the dry ingredients and whisk. You will have a runny, creamy batter, similar to a waffle batter.

6. Pour the batter into the sheet pan and bake for about 15 minutes. The cake will not be soft to the touch anymore, and it will smell like baked cake.

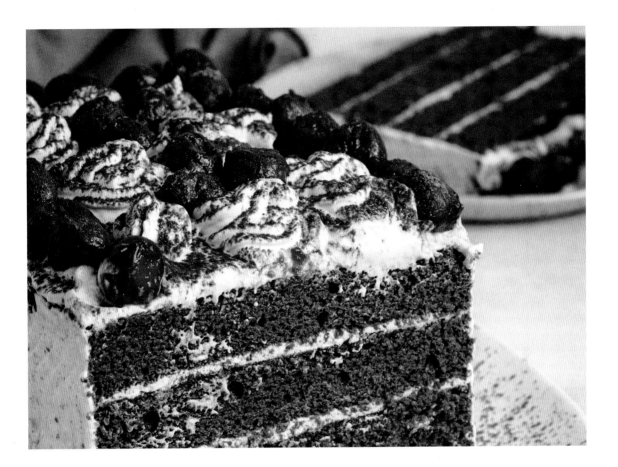

7. Take the sheet pan out and allow it to completely cool before assembling.

8. In the meantime, make the mascarpone and coconut cream. Add all the ingredients to a bowl and whisk with an electric mixer on high speed until the cream thickens and forms stiff peaks. Store it in the fridge until you are ready to assemble the cake.

9. To assemble the cake, cut the cake into four equal parts. Carefully lift one of the pieces with a spatula and arrange it on a platter. Add a layer of cream and then continue with the rest of the layers of cake and cream. With a big knife, even the rough edges. Top with a layer of cream and decorate as you wish. For a little bit of red, you can dust your cake with aronia berry or beetroot powder or simply use cacao or carob powder.

10. It is best is to store the cake in the fridge overnight before serving. It can be kept in the fridge for up to 3 days.

NOTE: If you can't have cacao, you can replace it with carob powder.

TIP: This can easily become a delicious tiramisu if you add some liquor and espresso to the batter and make the cream using raw eggs, like a traditional mascarpone cream for tiramisu.

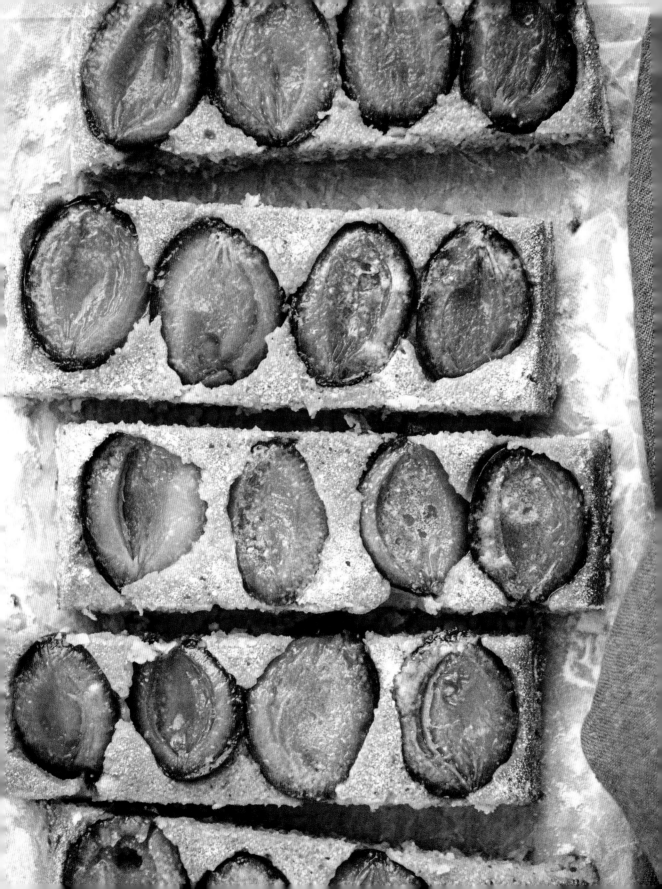

UPSIDE-DOWN PLUM COFFEE CAKE

If plums are in season, this cake is a must-make. It's very easy to put together but makes such a delicious and satisfying sweet treat.

Preparation time:
30 minutes

Cooking time:
20–25 minutes

Serves:
10

10 medium plums (more or less depending on the size)

1 teaspoon coconut oil

1–2 teaspoons inulin powder, plus more for dusting

½ cup (120 g) coconut cream

4 tablespoons (64 g) hazelnut butter

1 teaspoon local or raw honey or yacon syrup

2 pastured eggs

½ cup (40 g) shredded coconut

½ cup (60 g) tigernut flour

½ cup (52 g) almond flour

1 teaspoon baking powder

1 teaspoon pure vanilla extract or ¼ teaspoon vanilla powder

Zest of 1 organic lemon

¼ teaspoon salt

1. Preheat the oven to 350°F (180°C, or gas mark 4).

2. Wash the plums well, pat dry, and slice in half, removing the pit.

3. Prepare a shallow rectangular or square glass, ceramic, or stoneware baking dish with a similar volume to the one I used: approximately 7 × 11 inches (18 × 28 cm). A shallow dish will make it possible to flip the cake upside down. If the edges are too high, you won't be able to do it, but you can portion it in the dish and take it out slice by slice. A ceramic or stoneware round tart dish can also be used, but it will make portioning the cake more complicated. Generously coat it with coconut oil.

4. Arrange the plum halves, cut-side down, as many as you can fit in your baking dish. Dust 1 or 2 teaspoons of inulin powder on top of them.

5. In a big bowl, whisk the coconut cream, hazelnut butter, honey, and eggs until well combined and creamy.

6. Add the rest of the ingredients, one by one, and fold them in with a spatula.

7. Add the batter on top of the plums and level with a spatula.

8. Bake for about 20 minutes on a cake setting or a little more on a normal oven setting. The cake is ready when it is no longer soft to the touch and the edges start getting golden brown. The smell will guide you.

9. Remove the baking dish from the oven and let it cool for about 5 to 10 minutes. With a knife, make sure the edges are not sticking to the dish. With the help of a flat surface, like a cutting board, turn the cake upside down. The cake has to be still warm when you do this.

10. Let it cool completely and dust with inulin powder. Portion and serve.

PUMPKIN PIE SPICE LATTE

Bring your average-day hygge up a notch with this delicious, grounding, warming, and comforting pumpkin pie spice latte. It's perfect for the colder season or any day you feel like a pick me up.

Preparation time:
5 minutes

Cooking time:
5 minutes

Makes:
1 latte

½ cup (120 ml) hemp milk, homemade (page 33) or store-bought

2 tablespoons (30 g) coconut cream

1 heaping tablespoon (13 g) baked sweet potato, or more if you want a creamier and thicker texture

1 espresso (you can make it a double if you want something strong)

1 teaspoon hazelnut butter

½ teaspoon local or raw honey (or use a compliant sweetener, such as inulin powder, monk fruit, or yacon syrup and adapt to your desired sweetness)

Pinch of vanilla powder

¼ teaspoon pumpkin pie spice mix to your taste or use a mix of cinnamon and a pinch of nutmeg or ⅛ teaspoon licorice powder

1. Warm up the hemp milk, coconut cream, and sweet potato in a saucepan (don't worry about texture; it will all mix up in the blender). If you want a cold latte, there's no need to warm up ingredients.

2. Make the espresso (it can be a double if you want) and add all the ingredients in a high-powered blender. Mix and serve immediately.

3. I love adding licorice powder to my latte.

ALMOND THUMBPRINT COOKIES

The idea for these almond thumbprint cookies came after I tasted a (sugar-loaded) almond cake while in Denmark, where marzipan is king. If you don't know already, marzipan is actually a blanched almond paste mixed with sugar and sometimes with egg whites. So, a mix of almond butter, almond flour, and a compliant sweetener will give these cookies that marzipan flavor. To intensify the flavors, use a good-quality almond extract. I had these cookies with me during a road trip to Copenhagen, and they were such a treat.

Preparation time:
30 minutes

Cooking time:
20 minutes

Makes:
22 cookies

2 pastured eggs

1 cup (115 g) millet flakes (or just use almond flour only)

1 cup (104 g) plus 2 tablespoons (14 g) almond flour

4 tablespoons (56 g) coconut oil, room temperature

4 tablespoons (64 g) white almond butter (made with blanched almonds)

2 teaspoons local or raw honey, yacon syrup, or another preferred sweetener

2 tablespoons (28 ml) rose water

½ to 1 teaspoon almond extract (depending how much you love this flavor)

2 teaspoons pure vanilla extract (or vanilla powder or seeds from a pod; be generous if you like the vanilla flavor)

Zest of 1 big organic lemon (or from 2 small ones)

Pinch of salt

22–25 blanched almonds, whole

1 tablespoon (15 g) inulin powder

1. Preheat the oven to 350°F (180°C, or gas mark 4) and prepare a baking sheet.

2. Beat the eggs lightly in a small bowl.

3. In a big bowl, mix the millet flakes and almond flour. Add the coconut oil, almond butter, honey, rose water, almond extract, vanilla, lemon zest, salt, and beaten eggs and combine. Start mixing everything with your hands until you get a sticky dough.

4. Take about 1 tablespoon (15 ml) of dough and shape it into a ball. Add to the baking sheet. Repeat, making sure you leave some space in between.

5. Take one almond and gently press it in the middle of a dough ball. Repeat until you make all the cookies. I get about 22 cookies from this quantity.

6. Bake for about 20 minutes until golden brown. Let them cool down and dust them with inulin powder. You can eat them immediately, store them in the fridge for a day, or freeze them.

NOTES: You can use the same dough but make another filling—like a sugar-free homemade jam. To make these cookies, I use a baking sheet with holes, so time might vary depending on the type of pan you will use.

SWEET POTATO PIE

The quintessential holiday treat, the traditional sweet potato pie comes with at least 1 cup (200 g) of added sugar. This is a healthier version, but as delicious and satisfying. If you want to lower the carbohydrate load, use the Easy Keto Pie Crust, Without Eggs from page 68 instead.

Preparation time:
40 minutes

Cooking time:
30 minutes

Serves:
8

FOR THE CRUST:

1 cup (140 g) cassava flour

2 tablespoons (18 g) arrowroot flour

½ cup (56 g) coconut flour

1 tablespoon (12 g) monk fruit sweetener (I used golden)

¼ teaspoon salt

2 pastured eggs

1 teaspoon pure vanilla extract

⅔ cup (149 g) coconut oil, melted but not hot

FOR THE FILLING:

1⅔ cups (550 g) cooked sweet potato (about 2 medium potatoes; I cook them in an Instant Pot a day prior, but any cooking method would work)

4 tablespoons (60 g) coconut cream

2 pastured eggs

2 tablespoons (32 g) pecan butter

2–4 tablespoons (weight will vary) sweetener of choice (monk fruit is great for this)

1 teaspoon pure vanilla extract (or seeds scraped from a 2-inch [5 cm] vanilla pod)

¼ teaspoon sea salt

¼ teaspoon ground allspice or ¼ teaspoon nutmeg

1 teaspoon cinnamon

FOR SERVING (optional):

Whipped coconut cream

1. Preheat the oven to 350°F (180°C, or gas mark 4). Prepare a pie dish by greasing it with olive, coconut, or avocado oil.

2. Combine the flours, sweetener, and salt in a food processor.

3. Add the eggs, vanilla, and coconut oil and process on high until everything gets mixed together and forms a dough.

4. Take the dough out of the bowl and start kneading it. Shape the dough in a ball and leave it for 5 minutes to rest.

5. Prepare a work surface with two parchment papers and a rolling pin. Flatten the ball out on the bottom parchment paper, spreading it into a round. Add the parchment sheet on top and start rolling with a pin until you get a sheet about ¼ inch (6 mm) thick. The dough will crack a little bit on the edges, but it's easy to stick back together. Peel the top parchment paper off and carefully flip the dough on the top of the pie dish. At this point, some of the edges might fall off, but don't worry, they are very easy to stick back together. Fix the dough wherever it is broken and remove the excess edges. Let it rest in the fridge while you are making the filling.

6. To make the filling: Add all the ingredients to a food processor and combine until creamy.

7. Fill the pie dish with the sweet potato filling and bake for about 30 minutes. The edges should be golden brown and the top set and golden. Let slightly cool before serving or even better, refrigerate for a few hours.

8. Serve it as is or with a dollop of whipped coconut cream.

AVOCADO CHOCOLATE CHIP COOKIES WITH HAZELNUTS (and Cookie Dough)

Bake these cookies for 10 minutes or eat the dough with a spoon. It's your choice. Either way, if you love chocolate and hazelnuts, you are in for a treat. You can also use this dough as a chocolate cream filling for cakes, in which case don't add the coconut flour and the chocolate chips. If you are watching your carb intake, you can rejoice because these cookies are keto friendly.

Preparation time:
15 minutes

Cooking time:
10 minutes

Makes:
15 small cookies

1 cup (112 g) coarse hazelnut flour (grind the hazelnuts in a food processor, to a coarse flour)

1½ ripe avocados, medium size (2 if they are small)

¼ cup (20 g) raw cacao powder

3 tablespoons (48 g) hazelnut butter

3 tablespoons (36 g) monk fruit or another compliant sweetener

1 teaspoon baking powder

1 teaspoon pure vanilla extract (vanilla powder or vanilla pod can be used)

1 tablespoon avocado oil, MCT oil, or extra-virgin olive oil

1 tablespoon (7 g) coconut flour

Pinch of Himalayan pink salt or sea salt

⅓ cup (58 g) dark chocolate chips or chopped dark chocolate, above 85% cacao

More sea salt flakes for finishing

1. Preheat the oven to 350°F (180°C, or gas mark 4). Line a baking sheet with parchment paper (it also works without if you prefer).

2. Grind 1 cup (135 g) of raw hazelnuts in a food processor until you get coarse flour, about the size of rice (the cookies have crunch and texture from the bigger pieces of hazelnuts). Remove from the food processor and measure out 1 cup (112 g).

3. Add all the ingredients (minus the chocolate chips and the ground hazelnuts) to the food processor and process until well mixed, but don't overdo it. You will get a thick paste. Add the ground hazelnuts and pulse a few times to combine.

4. Add most of the chocolate chips (keep a few for decoration) and incorporate them with a spatula.

5. Take about 1 tablespoon (15 g) of the dough and shape into a ball and then gently flatten the balls out with a spatula.

6. Bake for 10 minutes. Sprinkle sea salt flakes on top and let them cool down to set (they are soft when out of the oven).

7. Remove them from the baking sheet with a spatula.

CHESTNUT CREPES WITH STRAWBERRIES AND PISTACHIOS

Crepes have always been my favorite sweet treat. I learned to make crepes when I was 10 years old, and I had to relearn how to make them lectin-free. So far, my favorite lectin-free crepes are made with chestnut flour. The texture is very similar to normal crepes, and the taste is even better. Chestnut flour is naturally sweet and full of flavor. You can use the basic recipe for any fillings you like, both sweet and savory.

Preparation time:
15 minutes

Cooking time:
30 minutes

Makes:
6 crepes

FOR THE CREPES:

2 pastured eggs

1 cup (235 ml) hemp milk, homemade (page 33) or store-bought

1 cup (112 g) chestnut flour

2 tablespoons (28 ml) sparkling water

1 tablespoon (15 ml) avocado oil

Zest of 1 organic lemon

Pinch of salt

Coconut oil for the pan

Optional: 2 tablespoons (28 ml) rose water

FOR SERVING:

3–4 tablespoons (32 to 64 g) hazelnut or pistachio butter (or a mix of both)

1 cup (145 g) fresh strawberries, sliced

½ cup (60 g) chopped pistachios

4 tablespoons (32 g) grated dark chocolate

1. Add all the ingredients for the crepes to a high-powered blender and mix until everything is smooth.

2. Warm a crepe pan or nonstick pan on medium heat and add a tiny bit of coconut oil to the pan.

3. Start cooking the crepes by adding about ¼ cup (60 ml) of batter to the pan, making sure the batter covers the entire pan as quickly as possible. Cook for about 2 minutes on the first side.

4. When the edges are cooked and the batter is no longer liquid on top, it's time to flip it. You can use a spatula to carefully peel the edges off and turn the crepe, or you can flip it like a chef. Please check tutorials online if you want to learn how. It's actually super fun.

5. Repeat with each crepe and pile them up on a plate.

6. Drizzle some nut butter on each crepe, add a few slices of strawberries and chopped pistachios, and fold them in triangles. Arrange them on a platter, drizzle more nut butter on top, garnish with slices of strawberries, sprinkle on some more pistachios and grated dark chocolate, and serve.

7. Refrigerate for a few hours before eating. Store in the fridge for up to 3 days.

HOW TO MAKE VEGAN CREPES

You would be surprised, but these crepes will work fine without eggs. Just mix flour, a liquid, and flavorings to get a crepe batter consistency and cook them as usual.

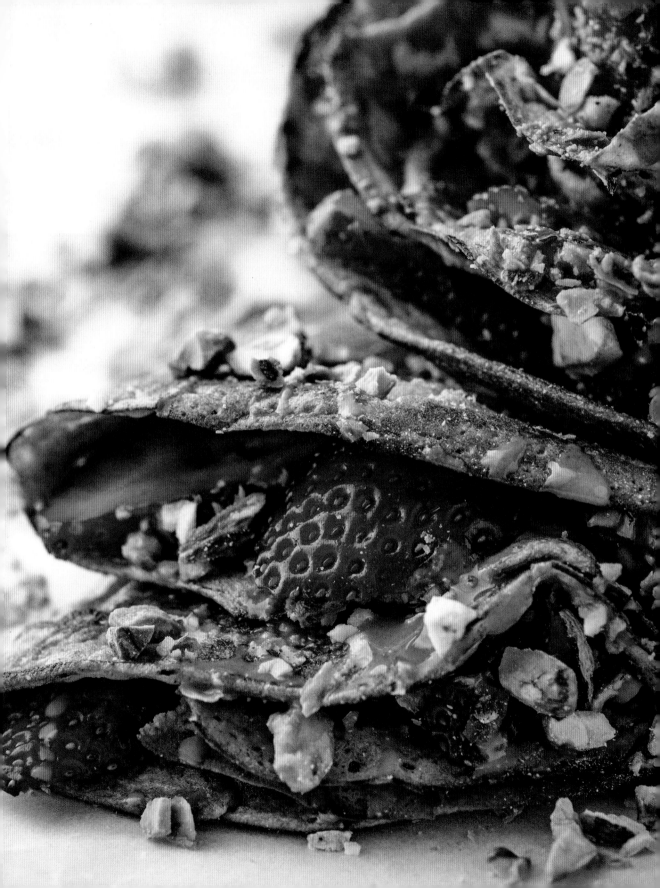

ABOUT THE AUTHOR

Claudia Curici is an Integrative Nutrition Health Coach and the founder of Creative in My Kitchen, a food and lifestyle blog where she writes about her health journey and posts original recipes that are always low-lectin, gluten-free, and sugar-free. She is the author of *The Living Well Without Lectins* cookbook, a printed collection of 125 lectin-free delicious recipes informed by her love of healthy food and decades of traveling and living on different continents.

After traveling and living around the world, Claudia started to feel like her health was declining in her late 30s, especially after she moved to the United States. While traditional medicine didn't have an answer for her and dismissed her symptoms and weight-gain as simply age-related hormonal fluctuations, she never stopped looking for answers.

Claudia first heard of lectins in July 2017 when she read an interview with Dr. Steven Gundry, the author of The Plant Paradox, about healthy foods that might make us sick. She started a lectin-free lifestyle and, since then, most of her symptoms have been resolved - and she lost the extra 25 pounds she gained in her late 30s.

On her blog, Creative in My Kitchen, and in her two cookbooks, she shares her everyday experiments with food, her joy of cooking tasty, nutritious and beautiful meals for herself and her family, and her health journey with others on the same path.

Claudia founded her blog while living in Dallas, Texas and now lives and creates from different places in Europe, including Romania and Denmark.

Follow Claudia on Instagram at @creativeinmykitchen for daily food inspiration.

ACKNOWLEDGMENTS

While my first book, *The Living Well Without Lectins Cookbook* was created in Dallas, Texas, this book was created part in Denmark, part in Romania. With social interactions reduced to a minimum during the pandemic, my main support during this time was my husband, Christian and my parents. Many of the recipes were brought to life while my husband and I were working on renovating our summerhouse in Denmark. Because one has to eat healthy, no matter what, right? Living in such a beautiful place, in the middle of nature, but also in need of easy and quick meals, inspired me to create simple and light recipes.

When we moved to Romania for the winter, my parents helped me create a studio space where I could store all of my pantry items and photography equipment. Living with my parents during the colder season inspired me to create family meals that are nourishing, grounding and delicious.

My main goal was to create dishes that anyone would eat without feeling they are on a diet. All the recipes in this book were tested by my husband and my parents and some of our friends and extended family. Usually, a recipe makes the book when people who are not on a diet love it. That's my ultimate test. Real food, made with seasonal, local and whole ingredients, should never be labeled as diet food.

I am beyond grateful for the support, guidance, encouragement and love I received from my husband, parents, friends and the community built around my social media channels and website. Without them, this book will not be possible.

Special thanks to Dr. Steven Gundry and to Lanee Neil, who have always been so supportive of my work. Grateful for the very special endorsements I got for my first cookbook from two of the people I admire the most in the health and wellness space: Dr. Terry Wahls and Dr. Will Cole.

Last but not least, I am grateful for the guidance and support of the Quarto team who helped me create this cookbook, and for their trust in me. Before working with them, I had no idea how much time, work, dedication, attention to detail, talent and team work are needed for making a cookbook.

INDEX

Note: Page references in *italics* indicate recipe photographs.